Sports Massage for Peak Performance

Sports Massage

for Peak Performance

GREGORY PIKE

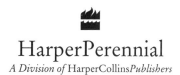

HarperPerennial
A Division of HarperCollinsPublishers

HarperCollins books may be purchased for educational, business, or sales promotional use. For information please write: Special Markets Department, HarperCollins Publishers, Inc., 10 East 53rd Street, New York, NY 10022.

FIRST EDITION

Designed by Laura Lindgren

Library of Congress Cataloging-in-Publication Data
Pike, Gregory, 1971–
    Sports massage for peak performance / by Gregory Pike. — 1st ed.
      p.   cm.
    Includes bibliographical references and index.
    ISBN 0-06-095167-2
    1. Massage therapy. 2. Sports physical therapy.   I. Title.
RC1226.P55   1997
615.8'22'088796—dc21   97-5528

97 98 99 00 01 ❖/RRD 10 9 8 7 6 5 4 3 2 1

Contents

Introduction

Welcome to *Sports Massage for Peak Performance*. This book was created to let you, the athlete, do better in your sport. As an athlete you place special demands on your body. You must make quick movements, some that are jarring, extreme, and repetitive, over long periods of time. You need extreme and unusual range of motion. Your muscles must generate great force within a short time. You need to be able to coordinate complex movements using many different muscles, and to be able to change direction or movements suddenly. In order to accomplish such things better than your competitors and without injuring yourself, you train and prepare in special ways, get proper nutrition and rest, and do other things that nonathletes don't do.

In recent years, as athletes have become more sophisticated and dedicated, they have discovered additional ergogenic aids—tools to improve performance and to find the winning edge—such as visualization, meditation, and stretching, for instance. One of the newest of these ergogenic techniques is massage. Massage is a tool. It is used to produce stress relief and body awareness, and to improve muscle efficiency, movement, and circulation. It can aid in rehabilitation from an injury, and it can help prevent injuries. Massage is accomplished by using a part of the massager's body—

hand, forearm, elbow, knee, even foot—to touch the recipient's body. It has been around since ancient times. Depictions of it are found in ancient Greek paintings, and it is described in ancient Indian and Chinese manuscripts. It has been used for many purposes, both physical and spiritual.

Massage includes virtually any form of bodywork from many different cultures. This includes shiatsu (a Japanese type of finger pressure on body lines of energy), polarity (light touch to balance electromagnetic energy), Trager (relaxation by repetitive body-loosening motions), rolfing (repositioning of how the body is held through intense manipulation), tu-na (a Chinese massage similar to shiatsu), and many, many others. The type of massage traditionally used in the United States and Europe—and the one we will use in this book, unless otherwise noted—is Swedish massage. It affects the soft tissues, such as muscles, tendons, and fascia (a connective tissue that encases organs, muscles, and other body structures), and the circulatory system (lymph and blood). It consists of five strokes: effleurage (long strokes), petrissage (deeper strokes), friction, vibration, and tapotment (rhythmic tapping), mostly carried out with the massager's hands and forearms.

Swedish massage involves physical manipulation. It does not depend on energy systems, the subject's receptive state of mind, spiritual theories, or nonphysical properties. Because it is hands-on work and it is systematic, it fits in well with the Western scientific approach. It is used in hospitals for physical therapy, rehabilitation, and to prevent bedsores in bedridden and paralyzed patients; it is used in spas for relaxation and for stress relief; it is used in offices for repetitive overuse injuries—carpal tunnel syndrome, low-back problems, and headaches. It is also increasingly used in sports.

Actually, massage has been used in America in some sports for decades. Early in this century, American athletes used sports massage to help them become the envy of the world by their accomplishments. When you think of a boxer in the locker room, you think of him getting a good "rubdown" from his trainer before the fight. The basic stroke was tapotment or pounding with the fists. This enabled the fighter to remain loose and warm and to get to the ring in peak form. Baseball pitchers, because of the specialized nature of their skill, its repetitiveness, and the extreme risk of damage and injury to the shoulder capsule, discovered the benefits of postperformance massage long ago out of necessity. A serious decline in performance would have been immediately obvious and ended their careers. The trainers used jostling, stretching, cramp release, and ice massage to prevent swelling and to help the pitchers come back quicker. In Europe, sports massage was used far more widely. In their quest for prestige and Olympic gold medals, Eastern-bloc teams in sports from gymnastics to weight lifting made massage a regular part of their training regimens. A friend of mine who played basketball in Germany in the seventies and eighties told me how he and his teammates got massages after every practice and game. He felt that massage had helped him prolong his career and avoid injuries that would have affected him to this day. However, the wide use of massage in sports took much longer to catch on in the United States.

The sports massage resurgence got a great boost here in America when a massage therapist by the name of Jack Meagher wrote the book *Sports Massage* in 1980. Around the same time in Chicago, Robert K. King, Jim Hackett, and others started teaching and writing about sports massage and began using it with marathon runners. They have gone on to work with such professional teams as the Chicago Bears, Bulls, and Blackhawks and have made sports massage an important part of the curriculum at their Chicago School of Massage.

Since the seventies, gradually more and more professional teams and championship athletes have begun incorporating massage into their training routines. The New York Giants, the New York Islanders, the New York Knicks' Patrick Ewing, and the U.S. Open tennis tournament are just a few examples. The American Massage Therapist Association has recently started giving out a certification in sports massage and continues to develop the criteria. Many massage therapists now advertise the ability to perform sports massage, although the skill is still so new and unstandardized that there is no guarantee of quality.

The strokes and techniques of sports massage come from Swedish massage, but the purpose of sports massage is to optimize the human body for a particular sport. The sports massage therapist focuses on the body parts used by the athlete in his or her sport, and the type of massage differs according to the intention: pre-event, post-event, and maintenance. The purpose of pre-event massage is to prepare the athlete for competition; post-event massage is used to help cool down and jump-start the healing process in the athlete after competition; maintenance massage works the body in between events to keep it functioning at a peak training level.

Unfortunately, as important and essential a tool as sports massage has become, many athletes still don't have access to a qualified sports massage therapist for reasons of expense and/or availability. This book is designed to bring the techniques of sports massage to every athlete. No previous training or special equipment is needed. Many of the strokes, exercises, and work-outs can be performed by the athlete on himself. Others can be performed with a training partner. All you need is dedication, perseverance, and prac-tice. Basic techniques and theories are given in the opening chapters and sports-specific routines follow. You will begin to experience the benefits almost immediately: you will learn about your body and how it works; your body will function more efficiently when you play your sport; you'll avoid injury because you'll be more flexible; and your tissues will be getting more nutrients and be able to better rid themselves of exercise-generated toxins. Put simply, you'll feel and perform better.

KEY POINTS:
1. Sports have become more arduous and competitive.
2. Successful athletes are using ergogenic aids to achieve their goals.
3. Massage is an ergogenic aid that has been around for ages.
4. Massage incorporates many types of bodywork.
5. Massage has been used successfully in sports to help athletes excel in Europe, Asia, and America.
6. Sports massage is made up of pre-event, post-event, and maintenance massages.

EXERCISE

The purpose of this exercise is to get you familiar with the body areas and to learn to place your hands on these body areas in a way that's comfortable for you.

1: Place your hands over all parts of your body. Try to feel how the hand fits to different body parts or areas, and incorporate those hand positions so they run together. When you find a good position for your hand, try to cover the area a different way to see if it feels better.

2: Start with your right hand on your left hand. Place your hand on the top, bottom, and both sides. Move to the wrist and repeat the top, bottom, and sides. Go to the forearm, upper arm, shoulder. Repeat on the other arm. Now, go to the forehead, jaw, face, temples, top of the head, back of the head, underneath the back of the head to the back of the neck, between the neck and shoulders, down the front of the body, up the opposite side to the armpits, down the back, to the butt, hips, thighs, back of the thigh, knee, around the lower leg, and all parts of the foot.

3: Now try your own sequence.

4: Rub or shake the areas briskly, as if you were warming them up.

Do you see how each time got easier as you got more in touch with your body? You may feel better from just frictioning—pressing into and moving the finger(s) back and forth—your body. Eventually you will find the method that works best for you and gets your entire body warm.

The aim of this exercise is to get you to sense your body through and with your hands, to progressively awaken your massage skills.

ONE

The Muscles

Before we get to sports massage, let's take a closer look at the objects of massage—muscles. Place your forearm on a table or leg, palm up, and relax your hand. With your other palm, press down just before the elbow of your upturned wrist. You'll notice that your fingers curl in. You have just discovered a principle whereby you are able to move your body.

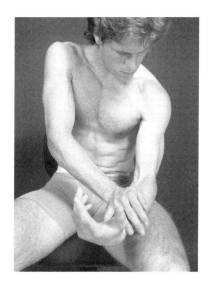

There are over 400 voluntary muscles in the human body. They take up 40 to 50 percent of total body weight and have a lined appearance, also known as "striated." They consist of bundles of fibers wrapped by connective tissues like wires in a cable. The muscle fibers run the entire length of the muscle, connecting to a tendon on each end. When you want to move, your brain sends a signal down the spinal chord, out a spinal nerve, and into the muscle, telling it to contract. The contraction pulls both the connective tissue surrounding the muscle and the tendon attached to the bone. The bone moves when the force of the muscle contraction through the tendon pulls on it.

Striated muscles are broken down into three types: slow twitch (type 1), intermediate (type 2a), and fast twitch (type 2b). The classifications are based on the length of time, amount of force, and the number of repetitions that it takes to tire the muscle (or use up the short-term energy available to the muscle). Every person has a different mixture of the three types, based on genetics. The good news is that you can change the mixture somewhat through training, making your 2a muscle fibers more like type 1 or like type 2b. Elite marathon runners usually have more type 1 fibers, which are important for endurance and repetitive movements over a long period of time. Elite sprinters usually have more type 2b fibers, important for explosive, powerful movements. Middle-distance runners may have more type 2a fibers.

For muscles to operate at top efficiency, they must be structurally sound. Any blockage, like a cyst or scar tissue, will cause the muscles to lose force or the force will act differently than usual. This is often a cause of tendinitis (inflammation of the tendon) or tenosynovitis (inflammation of the sheath surrounding the tendon). If muscles are undernourished they cannot put out maximum force or operate efficiently over long periods. For example, long-distance runners have worked out highly specialized dietary techniques, like carbo-loading and intake of electrolytes during races. Improperly developed muscles can cause strain on related muscles or improper body alignment, either of which can cause injury. An overdeveloped pectoralis major muscle (chest muscle) can cause a person to hunch forward, for example, which would be disastrous for a tennis player.

Muscles that are improperly warmed up won't have full range of motion, and force output will be diminished. To prove this to yourself try to imagine running a marathon as the first thing you do when getting out of bed. Lack of stretching can cause muscles to shorten, resulting also in loss of range of motion and injury. Gymnasts, who must have full range of motion for their sport, make stretching an integral part of their training regimen. Muscles that are too tense divert blood supply and cause the athlete distracting discomfort. Performance jitters can cause a figure skater to miss moves they routinely can do in practice.

It is the elite athlete's job to make certain that his or her muscles are in peak condition: properly trained, fed, stretched, warmed up, and ready to produce. At the level of world-class competition, native talent and genetic gifts are presupposed. Willpower, dedication, understanding of the sport and one's own body, and the discipline to prepare in whatever way is necessary, decide who wins the gold medal.

THE MUSCLE GROUPS AND WHAT THEY DO
The Foot Muscles

These small but important muscles are located on the bottom of the foot and are used to absorb shock and transfer force up the leg, to stabilize and propel the body, and to give the foot structure. These muscles run from the heel to the toes and are important for virtually every sports movement. (Think how hard it is to stand up a doll that is anatomically correct but lacks these muscles.)

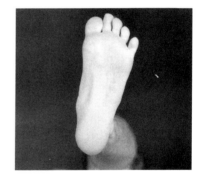

The Calf Muscles

These muscles run from near the knee to the heel on the back of the leg. The gastrocnemius muscle is closer to the skin while the soleus muscle lies underneath. They enable you to press your foot off the ground and point your foot. Obviously, these muscles are crucial for walking, running, and jumping.

Outside Lower Leg Muscles

Called the peroneal group, these three muscles run from below the knee into the foot. They pull

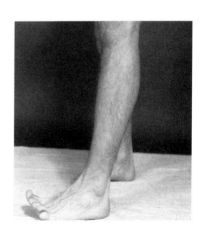

the outside of the foot outwards and upwards when you walk, run, or jump. They help the foot avoid turning in and spraining the ligaments on the outside of the ankle.

Front Lower Leg Muscles

These are located on the outside of the shin or tibia bone. They run from below the knee to the foot. They raise the foot so that you do not trip over your toes, and they help cushion the shock of walking or running. This is where you will feel the pain of a shinsplint.

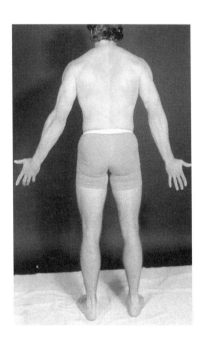

Back Thigh Muscles

Called the hamstrings, these three muscles run from the bony protuberances you sit on to the inside and outside of the lower leg bone. They enable you to kick your lower leg back and to raise your whole leg to the rear. The hamstrings are of particular importance to sprinters, swimmers, and any sport that requires running.

Front Thigh Muscles

These four muscles, called the quadriceps group, run from your hip to your knee. They enable you to kick forward, as with a soccer ball or football, and let you raise your body by straightening your knee, as when walking up steps.

Inside Thigh Muscles

These are the groin muscles, which run from the upper inner thigh down to the inside of the lower leg, below the knee. Called the abductors, they move the leg in the motion used for a breaststroke kick in swimming. Because these muscles are not the biggest prime movers, athletes often don't stretch them properly—which can result in groin tightness or pulls.

Butt Muscles

Known as the gluteus maximus, they are the major muscles pulling the body up in a weight lifter's squat or even getting up out of a chair. They also extend the lower leg from the hip, enabling the athlete to push the body forward by pushing off the leg.

Hip Muscles

Located in the area bordered by the back and front pockets of your pants, these muscles help you walk, stand up on one leg, and lift the leg up to the side, as ballet dancers and martial arts practitioners do.

Stomach Muscles

The four major abdominal muscles are located from the rib cage down to the pelvis and out to the lower back on the sides. They enable you to pull your upper body down and forward and also rotate it side to side. They also help to transfer force from the lower body to the upper body, as in a tennis serve.

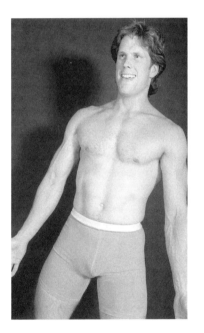

Lower Back

Located between the back ribs and the back of the pelvis, the quadratus lumborum helps you maintain erect posture and bend the upper body from side to side.

Center Back Muscles

The erectors and other muscles beneath them run from pelvis to head on either side of the spine. They help stabilize and rotate the trunk.

The Neck Muscles

These are located on the front, back, and sides of the neck. They run from the head to the shoulders; the back neck muscles are a continuation of the center back muscles. They stabilize and hold up the head, let you rotate it, and also pull it forward, sideways, and backwards. Most athletes who play contact sports—hockey, boxing, football, wrestling—need very strong, loose necks, and can easily injure these muscles.

Face and Head Muscles

These are on the face and the sides of the head. They move the jaw, enable you to make facial expressions, and help you talk. These muscles can also hold incredible amounts of tension and can result in temporomandibular joint (TMJ) problems and headaches, including migraines.

Shoulder Blade Muscles

These muscles are located on and all around the shoulder blade. They help hold the shoulder blades in place, and move them in all directions, even into the ribs, which are located under them. The four rotator cuff muscles are part of this group, and injuries to those are career-ending for pitchers, swimmers, wrestlers, and football players.

Chest Muscles

The pectorals are muscles that run along the front chest. These muscles are the prime movers when doing a push-up. The pectoralis major runs from the sternum out to the upper arm and the pectoralis minor runs from a part of the rib cage out to an anterior articulation of the scapula.

Upper Arm and Shoulder Muscles

The deltoids run from the shoulders to the outside of the upper arm, and enable you to do any shoulder movement. The trapezius run from the neck to the shoulders and down to the upper back, and enable you to shrug your shoulders. These muscles are very important for baseball players, gymnasts, tennis players, and football players.

Front Upper Arm Muscles

The biceps goes from the shoulder to the top of the forearm and the brachialis muscle goes from the mid-upper arm to the upper forearm. They let you pull your forearm up and turn your wrist inward, respectively.

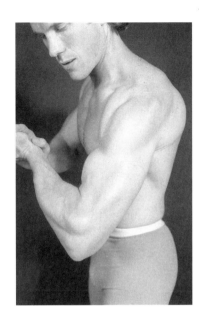

Back Upper Arm Muscles
Located on the back of the arm between the shoulder and the elbow, the triceps and extensors enable you to extend the elbow and are important for pitchers, boxers, tennis players, and any athletes who must use their upper arms.

Inside Forearm Muscles
The wrist flexors run from the elbow down into the hand, and enable you to flex the wrist and curl your fingers. These are used for more intricate and stabilizing movements—holding a baseball, pulling a trigger, holding a weight, etc. These muscles are the ones implicated in "golf elbow."

Outside Forearm Muscles
The wrist extensors run from the elbow down into the back of the hand. They balance the wrist flexors and allow you to extend the wrist and open the fingers. These fine muscles are easily injured from the forceful motions of certain sports like tennis and baseball. They are implicated in "tennis elbow."

The Hand Muscles
The muscles located in the hand help in the more intricate movements of the fingers and are crucial for grasping a baseball, golf club, or tennis racket, for rock climbing, etc.

While certain muscles are obviously crucial for certain athletes—for example, shoulder muscles and a football quarterback or baseball pitcher—the most basic sports movement is an almost unimaginably complex cooperation among virtually all your muscles. Take, for example, a right-handed quarterback who wants to throw a pass.

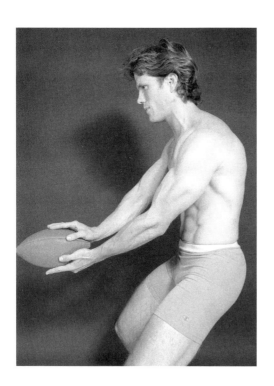
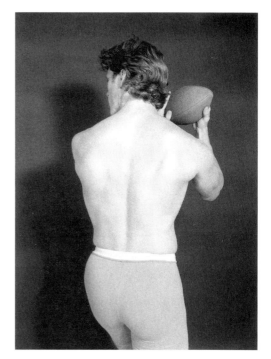

As the quarterback takes the snap from the center with his body parallel to the line of scrimmage, the ankle is dorsi-flexed, the knees are bent, the hips, spine, shoulders, and elbows are partially flexed. The left elbow is supinated (palm up) and the right elbow is pronated (palm down). After the snap, the athlete backpedals, his body perpendicular to the line of scrimmage. The arms go up behind him to his right ear. The feet plantar-flex to push off, the knee extends on the bent planted leg. The left leg abducts (pushes away) and the right leg adducts (pulls toward) as the legs cross-shuffle. The spine rotates the left shoulder forward and extends up. The head rotates to the left to spot his receivers. As the quarterback plants to throw the ball after the drop back, the right leg pushes off so that the ankle plantar-flexes again. The right knee extends, the right hip extends and externally rotates (meaning the thigh bone moves on the planted foot so that the body rotates to

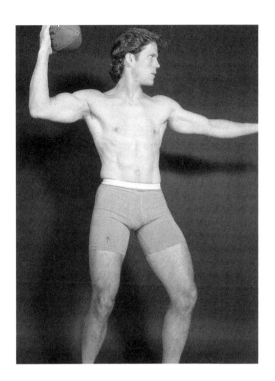
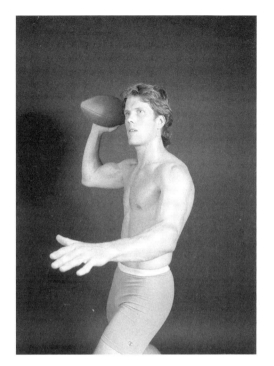

the left). The spine rotates slightly to the right and then explosively to the left. The forces of the lower body and trunk are transferred up to the right shoulder, which externally rotates slightly, then internally rotates and extends to throw the ball. The elbow also extends and the head rotates to the right to follow the thrown ball. The ankle of the left leg passively dorsi-flexes on the ground. The left knee and hip flexes as the front leg bends. The left arm is held out straight, pointing to the target. During the follow-through, the elbow of the right arm extends fully, the shoulder extends and internally and horizontally rotates to cross the body. The spine rotates to the left and flexes. The right hip extends and externally rotates. The right foot plantar-flexes, and the knee stays in extension as the weight is shifted from the right side of the body to the left.

This is only a sketchy, simplified kinematic study, but it gives a good idea of how many muscles and tendons are involved in a key sports movement. The major muscles involved in throwing the football include: triceps, deltoids, latissimus dorsi, the muscles along the spine, the four abdominals, the gluteals, the hamstring and quadriceps groups, the soleus, and gastrocnemius. If any of these muscles are underdeveloped, injured, not warmed up, or otherwise operating inefficiently, the ability of the passer will be effected negatively. When Troy Aikman, quarterback of the Dallas Cowboys, strained his calf muscles, he had to sit out games.

In the following chapters you will learn how to perform sports massage for particular sports, emphasizing the muscles most important to that sport. However, you should be aware of all the muscles you use and how you use them, and thereby develop a holistic approach to stretching, massage, and other body care.

KEY POINTS:

1. Muscles move the body by pulling on tendons that attach to bones.

2. Movement muscles are classified as slow, intermediate, and fast twitch (type 1, 2a, and 2b).

3. The movement muscles of the body can by classified in groups. The groups are: foot, calf, outside lower leg, front lower leg, back thigh, front thigh, inside thigh, butt, hip, stomach, lower back, center back, neck, face and head, shoulder blade, chest, upper arm and shoulder, front upper arm, back upper arm, inside forearm, outside forearm, hand.

4. A brief kinematic study of a quarterback throw illustrates the number of muscles involved in a simple movement.

EXERCISE: HAND STRENGTHENING

The purpose of this exercise is to strengthen the forearm muscles, the wrist, and the hands to prepare you for massage.

1: Hold your hands out in front of your body with the arms straight. The palms are down. Clench your hands as tight as you can and make a fist. Release and spread the fingers as wide as possible. Breathe out as

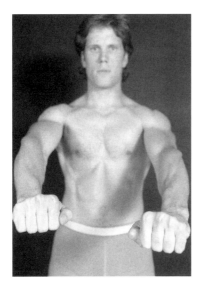 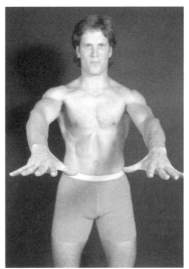

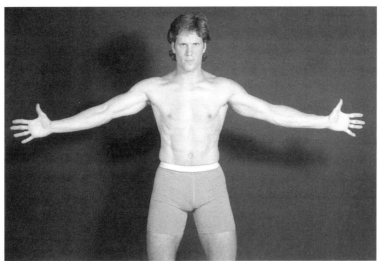

you grab and tense. Breathe in as you release and spread the fingers. Repeat till the muscles in the hand and wrist get tired or tight. Finish by loosening the muscles: shake out the wrists vigorously from side to side.

2: Hold the arms out to the side, palms facing frontward. Bring the fingers together, but keep them pointed out straight. Spread the fingers out wide so there is the greatest amount of space between each finger. Bring the fingers back together and repeat till the muscles get tired or

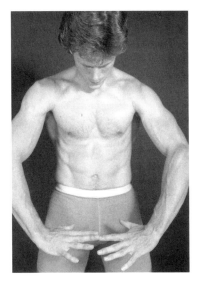

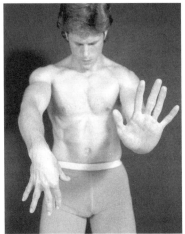

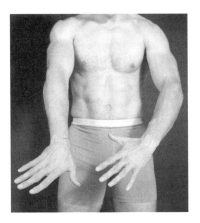

tight. Breathe with an even deep pace. Shake out the wrists to loosen the muscles.

3: Hold the arms out to the front. Turn the wrists slowly in large circles 10 times. Stop and circle 10 times in the other direction. Now do the same exercise, but this time tense the movements. Repeat the wrist circles in the other direction as you tense them. Breathe deeply and calmly with the movements. Shake out the wrists.

4: Hold the arms out in front with the palms down. Keeping the arms straight, bend the wrist up and down 20 times. Stop. Bend the wrist from side to side as you keep the arms still and straight. The wrists bend to the inside of the forearm and out to the outside of the forearm. Breathe calmly. Finish by shaking out the wrists.

The Basics of Sports Massage

WHEN *NOT* TO DO SPORTS MASSAGE

Now that you know what the body is, the next thing you should know is when not to do sport massage on it. In certain situations, massage can cause undesirable effects—hindering performance, spreading toxins or disease, or further complicating an injury. Do no work on yourself or someone else when:

1. They are under the influence of alcohol or drugs. (You might make it spread faster and throughout the subjects' system.)
2. They have a fever or are physically ill.
3. They have a disease that is currently contagious: poison ivy, skin rash, herpes, etc.
4. They have just eaten a full meal. (Massage hinders digestion, plus it feels uncomfortable.)

5. They are under treatment or treatments of cortisone. (This may weaken the bone structures, which may then be damaged by pressure.)
6. They are being treated with other medications. (Find out why they are using them. It may be for one of the above reasons.)
7. They are dehydrated.
8. They have a bone disease. (You may break their bones.)
9. They have cancer. (Massage may help spread the metastasized tissues to unaffected areas, thus spreading the cancer.)
10. They are in advanced stages of diabetes or cardiac condition (a recent heart attack or untreated blood pressure).

You may work on someone with the following problems but avoid the affected areas:
1. An open or draining wound.
2. Acute edema or inflammation.
3. Redness, heat, pain, loss of movement.
4. Bruises or lesions.
5. A slipped disk.
6. A cyst or tumor.
7. Keloid scar (raised, red growth).
8. Varicose veins.
9. A fractured bone.
10. Frostbite or burns.
11. Phlebitis (inflamed blood vessels), Burger's disease, or a blood clot.
12. Severe pain in the joints, bone, or muscle.

These lists may make you think that you should never touch anyone, but try not to be discouraged. Most of these warning signals are easily recognized, and if you're ever in doubt, just ask the subject. You can and should work on the areas surrounding the problem. An example would be an athlete who has a blister on the heel of his foot. You can still do sports massage on the bottom of the foot. Another example would be a bruise on the vastus lateralis (a quadriceps muscle on the outer part of the thigh). You may still work other parts of that muscle, but keep off the bruised area. If you locate any area that you are not sure about, *do not work on it!* It is also imperative that you let the person know if you discover a problem. They might not know they have something that needs to be checked out. For example, a blister on the foot of a marathon runner: he may be so pumped full of adrenaline he doesn't know his foot needs medical attention. Sports massage can help the body heal itself, but it is not the only or necessarily the best method for some injuries.

Sports massage takes a backseat to standard medical treatments in certain crucial situations. As a practitioner, you must try to recognize these situations and encourage the athlete to get the care he needs. One situation that you may come across is dehydration. In this case, the athlete needs medical care as soon as possible to avoid damage to organs, tissues, and the brain, or even death. Once he gets the proper care from a medical doctor and is okayed for a sports massage, you can continue. Among the situations that need immediate medical care are the following: seizures, coma, cardiac arrest, bone breaks, muscle tears, concussions, shock, and arterial bleeding. You should always know a number to call in case of an emergency.

KNOWING YOUR PARTNER

Before doing sports massage, it is important to know what type of person you are working on and the special considerations that must be given to him or her. People who may need special treatment in sports massage are seniors, children, people without a limb or body part, people with an artificial limb or body part, or any combination of the above. It is important to be sensitive to these people's needs. When massaging a senior (aged 65 +), it is important to start and finish lightly and gently. Their body will take more time to heal, change, and accept the bodywork. Their bones, muscles, heart, and the rest of their body may not take an intense, deep-pressure massage. One must be careful and cautious. For children, it is important to keep the massage light and short. Their young bodies are quick to heal and usually do so by themselves. The massage should just help and speed this process. For older children, some deep tissue work is good if they are very active and physical. The pressure of the deep tissue work is light. Adults, on the other hand, can take the deep pressure work. People without a body part can be massaged as usual with special care around the injured or missing body part. Ask the person what they want when you get to the body area in question. They are the ones who know it and how it feels. The same goes for artificial body parts. Each situation is specific to that person. It is also important to ask if the artificial limb has limited movement and cannot be placed or moved in a specific range of motion or plane. As a massager, you must consider all of the factors and modify your massage to those factors.

DOING SPORTS MASSAGE

So when do you do sports massage? You do sports massage on a person before and after competition. Prior to a competition, it is best to do the sports massage 15 to 45 minutes before the athlete will compete to help warm up muscle and connective tissue through friction and increased blood flow. The pre-event massage may be done up to four hours before the start of the event. After the competition, it is best to do the sports massage right after their personal cooldown routine. This massage will help drain toxins, replenish aching muscles, and invigorate and soothe the subject. A third type of massage is maintenance, to be performed between competitions. This deeper, more complete massage helps rehabilitate a major injury, rejuvenate after a strenuous workout or competition, and restore the body from tense and strained areas. The maintenance should be done no closer that 48 hours before a competition. The New York Giants had their maintenance sports massages done on Tuesdays and Thursdays to help heal before and after an game.

The Right Atmosphere

Sports massage is given in a relaxed manner. The surrounding space should be warm, safe, comfortable, and relaxing. The athlete should be sitting or lying down. Towels or a sheet are used for comfort and to keep the massage area clean. You should try to keep both hands on the person at all times. Your hands can be doing different things—one does a general stroke while the other is stationary, for instance. This gives you more control and is more comfortable and reassuring for the athlete.

Preparing to Massage

Some other things to consider are: keep your hands clean (wash your hands before and after massage if you can or use towel wipes) for cleanliness and safety; do not wear any jewelry (rings and watches) and keep your fingernails short to avoid scratching the skin; wear loose and professional clothing.

Before you begin you should stretch and warm up. Giving sports massage can be just as taxing as playing a sport, and you should approach it as such. Warm up your thighs, knees, shoulders, wrist, and hands (see pre-event massage to get some ideas). Remember to loosen your jaw and wrists.

Using the Correct Form

Form is important, as is your body alignment and body weight, which apply the force to massage the muscles. You should face the direction of the stroke. Your hips and shoulders should be parallel to each other. Use your legs, shift your weight, and push into the floor. Avoid pulling strokes—they're more tiring and stressful on you. Your wrists should be loose and straight when possible. If standing, do not lock your knees or elbows. Be careful of your thumbs, do not overwork or strain them. Lean your weight onto the person to help apply pressure. You do this to avoid fatiguing your own muscles and getting your own overuse injuries. Try to be as continuous and smooth as possible. Make the massage techniques and stretches flow. This takes practice, but you will improve as you become more comfortable. It will mark you as an accomplished sports massage practitioner. Do not worry at first if you forget any techniques. Just try to remember the core strokes and let them continuously flow out of you onto the athlete. Remember, you can always go back and do a particular stroke. Also, you should be aware of your own body's comfort and alignment. If your body is not comfortable, then your hands will communicate that to the athlete.

Breathing

Breathing is another important component of sports massage and an excellent gauge of how the massage is going. Correct breathing in sync with the strokes ensures that the massager will not get overtired from the work and that the subject will get full benefit from the massage. During the massage, both should breathe slowly and deeply into the lower abdomen and exhale evenly, slowly, and completely, as in the following exercise:

1: Place palms just below belly button, interlace fingers slightly, relax your throat and tongue, and breathe slowly in through your nose. Visualize the breath going down the body into the lower belly underneath your hands.

2: As the stomach extends, watch your fingers move away from each other. Hold the deepest point of the inhale for one second and then exhale through your mouth as if you were blowing out a candle. In doing so, relax the extended lower abdomen and watch your hands come together again. Then, at the point of the greatest exhale, hold the breath for one second.

3: Repeat this cycle 10 times and notice how you feel—energized and relaxed.

This breathing technique allows you to gain the optimal benefit from the pace of the strokes, helps get rid of carbon dioxide and tension, and brings more oxygen into the body and tissues.

The Importance of Feedback

Before the massage, the massager and the subject should discuss certain guidelines that will help increase the efficiency of the massage and improve enjoyment of it for both parties. First, the subject should ask himself how he feels (tired, cranky, anxious, excited, etc.), what his mental state is (happy, sad, stressed, etc.), and where he is tight and needs the most work, and communicate all this to the massager. Then the massager must consider this information and focus on the purpose of the massage. Why is it being given? This is a major concern when deciding how or what to do on the body. In general, massage is given to relax, but there are different kinds of relaxation. One is to still the mind and its racing thoughts; another is to loosen tight muscles. The pace, depth, type of stroke, and technique used are all variables to mix and match to achieve the desired effect. Throughout the massage, this type of feedback should continue. The feedback should consist of: "it feels good," "that's not comfortable," "not so deep," "stop," etc. He should tell you if it feels too deep or too light, if he feels any pain or discomfort, and if you are relieving the pain or discomfort. Monitor facial and body expressions. The subject's face and body should be relaxed, so if you cause a body part to flinch, you're working too fast or deep. He should let you do the work, should be relaxed and aware of what is happening inside his body. The more he holds tension or helps you raise that leg, the less benefit he will receive. He should breathe naturally, in and out. Make sure that he does not hold his breath.

A good way to understand how sports massage affects the body is to get one yourself. I regularly have a two-hour martial arts class in the morning and a strength-training session later in the day. My first sports massage was after these regular events. Unfortunately, I did not drink enough water afterward to help drain from my body the toxins released during exercise. The next day, I felt as if a train had hit me. I learned from that to drink plenty of water after a massage. And so should you.

THE THREE TYPES OF MASSAGE

Sports Massage falls into three categories: pre-event, post-event, and maintenance.

Pre-event

Pre-event massage is done before a competition or practice. Its objectives are to increase circulation, increase range of motion of the joints, decrease tightness and hypertonicity of major joints and muscles, and to relax and then invigorate the body to get it ready for the competition. It is to prepare the athlete to be optimally ready for their event and is an addition to the regular warm-up. The warm-up is an important part of athletic performance, as it helps you get ready for an event physiologically (oxygenates and flushes muscle) and psychologically (relaxes and energizes), and it helps avoid injuries. Athletes can also use this quality downtime to do breathing exercises, visualizations, or meditations.

Many athletes have had major or career-ending injuries from not warming up or improper warm-up. Certain overuse injuries can be avoided if the person properly warms up. The warm-up prepares an athlete to be ready at the start of the event, not 5 or 10 minutes into the event.

The pre-event sports massage is a nonspecific, general massage consisting of compression strokes, stretches, jostling, nonspecific friction, and range-of-motion techniques—things that you will learn further on in this book. The techniques focus on the major body parts and areas that the athlete will use during competition or practice. The pre-event massage should be done 15 to 45 minutes before the event or practice and should last up to 20 minutes. The massage should be done just before the athlete's usual, proper warm-up. If the athlete cannot give enough time, do what you can and just focus on the most important areas needed in the sport—the thighs, legs, and feet for a runner, for example. For a pitcher, it would be his pitching arm and trunk.

It is important in pre-event massage not to do deep work that requires time for the body to adjust. And the massage should not be painful. Keep it light, warming, upbeat, and rhythmical, not slow. Do not use ice or ice massage. And remember: no more than 15 to 20 minutes, no deep tissue, and nonspecific.

Post-event

Post-event massage is done after the event or practice. The goals are to relax tight muscles, decrease muscle soreness, facilitate faster recovery time, relieve cramping, increase lymphatic circulation and removal of postactivity metabolites, and relax the nervous system. It is an addition to the cooldown of the athlete, which brings the athlete down physiologically (relaxes hypertonic, or tight and wiry, muscle tension and decongests) and psychologically (relaxing) from the competition back to everyday life. This type of massage promotes cellular waste removal and replenishes the body. Cooldown is very important to avoid cramps, to prevent the pooling of blood in the lower extremities, to stretch and relax muscles, and to help the body begin the healing process for a quicker recovery. The post-event massage should last 20 minutes, but it may get up to 60 to 90 minutes for ultra-endurance events (marathons, biking, or Iron Man competitions). The postevent massage can also help prevent delayed onset muscle soreness (DOMS). DOMS is pain felt 8 to 24 hours after the exertion. The pain will peak at around 48 hours after the event and it will dissipate in a few days after that. DOMS is a form of acute inflammation and the symptoms are pain, swelling, reduced range of motion, and a decrease in strength and ability to perform. Post-event sports massage seems to be effective in decreasing DOMS if performed within two hours after stopping strenuous exercise.

The techniques that will be used here are compression strokes, jostling, stretches, cramp relief techniques, petrissages, shaking, and range-of-motion (ROM) techniques. (Again, you'll learn more about this later.) During the post-event massage, these questions can be helpful: "Where do you need the massage the most?" or "How does this feel?" to check depth. Key points to remember are: do not do deep tissue work, do not use heat, and do the massage only after the athlete has cooled down properly through a light workout and stretching. Do not work on suspected strains, sprains, cuts, bruises, blisters, or fractures. Work at a slow, relaxing pace. Take the athlete's shoes off for him. You are preparing the athlete to go home. Do not do anything painful.

Maintenance

Maintenance massage is done between events. Its objectives are to loosen tissue, to remove trigger points and knots, to decrease hypertonicity and tightness, to improve posture, to relax, or any other reason to get a deep tissue massage. This type of massage is not done the day before or after a major event because the body will need at least 48 hours to adjust to the body reconstruction. Think of maintenance as an overhaul of the body. This is the massage that everyone commonly thinks about: on a table, with oil or creme, and music. It does not have to be done with creme or oil. It does not have to be done on an expensive massage table or even with music. All these additions are nice, and I highly recommend them for that great massage. But in this book the maintenance massage will be shown on the ground or chair, without oil or creme, and with the clothes on. Maintenance massage uses all the stokes: effleurage, petrissage, vibration and tapotment, friction, myofascial, and any other technique that is used in massage. Maintenance massage commonly last between 30 to 90 minutes. Maintenance massage can be to the entire body or to just a body part or area. We'll cover this more completely later in the book.

KEY POINTS:

1. When not to do sports or any massage.
2. When not to work on a body part or area on someone.
3. Do sports massage on someone *only* if the person does not need immediate medical care.
4. Sports massage benefits the athlete the best when it is done 15 to 45 minutes before or after a competition.
5. Sports massage is broken down into three parts: pre-event, post-event, and maintenance.
6. The sports massage should be clean, safe, relaxing, and dry.
7. Feedback given to the massager: "stop," "that feels good," "that's not comfortable," and "not so deep."
8. Questions asked during the massage: "how does that feel?" and "is that deep enough?"
9. Watch the person's body for cues: tensing, holding the breath, wincing, sharp intake of the breath, and others. Alter your massage to their benefit.
10. Pre-event massage is done before an event, is an addition to the athlete's regular warm-up, and gets the body primed for competition.
11. Postevent massage is done after an event, is an addition to the athlete's cooldown, and helps the body recuperate from the event.
12. Maintenance massage is done between events and is an overhaul of the body.

EXERCISE 1

The purpose of this exercise is to see and feel how body parts move and to feel the relaxing/energizing affect of these movements.

1: Starting with your toes, move each of your joints in as many movements and directions as possible. Go from the toes to the ankles, to the knees, hips, spine, to the shoulder, elbow, forearm, wrist, fingers, neck (avoid rotation to the rear, which could hurt a disk between the vertebrae), and to the jaw.

2: Do all the motions in a controlled, slow, and relaxed manner. Breathe with all the motions. For example, breathe in as you drop your head back, breathe out as you drop the chin to your chest. Afterwards, feel how your body is relaxed and energized.

3: If you have a partner, do the same exercise, but move all their joints in different range of motions. The movements are slow, relaxed, cause no pain, are circular or straighter, or a combination of circular and straight. Start with the major joints like the hip, knee, shoulders, and arms first. Feel how heavy their relaxed body parts are. The movements should be smooth and they should not be helping in any way except relaxing. Have them breathe into the movements with slow, deep breaths.

4: Afterwards, ask about how their body feels. How do they feel emotionally. Are there any areas or range of motions that they liked or disliked? Which ones? Ask yourself the same questions after you do this to them. Also, is there any way that you could have done it better?

EXERCISE 2

The purpose of this exercise is to mentally relax the body. This type of relaxing is called an autogenic training exercise. Read all the instructions through first before trying it.

Note that it is preferable to use a hard surface rather than a soft bed. The reason for this is that the body must be in its most relaxed position on a hard floor in order not to hurt. The relaxed body will conform to the floor, while a tight body will feel pain because the body cannot relax completely. A soft bed will conform to your body so that your body does not have to relax and can stay tight. This is one reason why you can be sore after sleeping on a soft bed.

1: Lie on your back. We are going to relax the entire body. Afterward we will scan the body to find the tight and sore areas.

2: Relax the body by breathing into the body parts slowly and deeply. We will move up from the feet to the head, relaxing all our body parts. You can use other relaxing cues to have the body part relax. Feel heat and weight for kinesthetic. Hear soft peaceful music or other sounds for auditory. Smell a favorite smell like your favorite breakfast. See a peaceful scene or color. Even taste a favorite taste that reminds you to relax. Do any, all, or a combination of these to help the body parts to relax.

3: Start at the toes. Breathe in and out. Move to the feet, the ankles, the lower leg, the knees, the thighs, the hips, the trunk, the lower back, the abdominals, the chest, the middle and upper back, the shoulders and upper arms, the forearms, the wrist and hands, the fingers, up to the neck, the scalp, the jaw, the ears, the eyes, the nose, the mouth, the tongue, the forehead. Feel the relaxation all through your body. Stay with it and breathe in and out deeply.

4: After a few minutes, scan your body and search for those tight, painful areas. Are they in your neck, back, or elsewhere? These are the areas that you need to massage. These areas, called trigger points, are your chronic tense areas.

5: Now slowly get up and map the body. Mark down with Xs where you felt the tension. After a period of time, do this exercise again and see if the tense areas are still there or if you gained a few in your hectic daily life.

THREE

The Basic Strokes

Now let's outline the basic strokes. We'll look at what they are, how they are done, what they do to the body, when to do them, and which body parts they're used for. When doing any of these strokes or techniques, it is important to think about the depth (how light or deep the pressure) and frequency (how fast or slow).

If you are on the biggest part of the muscle, you can work on the surface, in the middle, or deep down into the muscle belly (areas of large muscle fiber). The depth of the stroke will determine which part you will be working on. In most strokes, light pressure is best. Light pressure lets the athlete get used to your touch and feel comfortable and safe with you. It will help relieve what you are focusing on by breaking apart the easy stuff and warming and loosening the harder stuff. To push your way in too deep too fast will make the muscles contract and not let you get in. The body will let you know when to go deep: the tissue warms, softens, and relaxes; the light pressure you are applying will want to sink into the muscle. It is then that you go deeper. It is amazing what can be done by making the muscles relax gradually instead of trying to force things. As you increase the pressure, remember to use your body weight and not your muscle strength. It feels better to both you and the subject, and you can do more work by not tiring out your smaller muscles.

Some people think that the sports massage has to be painful. It should not be. It is extremely important to let good sense be your guide. You must learn to judge the athlete's pain sensitivity, and know your reasons for working on a particular area. The ability to do this is gained through experience, by working on many people. As a beginner, try to err on the conservative side. At least you won't be doing any harm or making the athlete uncomfortable.

The purpose of the massage will determine the frequency of the stroke. A slow stroke will relax and sedate the athlete, which is the goal of the postevent sports massage or at the end of the maintenance massage. The slow frequency will soothe, and get you through the superficial tissues to the deeper ones by making the tissues mushy. A fast frequency will invigorate and tone the muscle. A medium frequency will do a little of both, and the effects will not be as extreme. Sometimes you can combine different frequencies so that you can vary a stroke to get different and exciting results. As you gain experience, try different frequencies with different strokes to vary your massage.

Effleurage

Effleurage are long, light strokes. They are executed by applying light pressure with the palm of your hand while moving it over the surface of the skin. Effleurage is done as a beginning or transition stroke on a large area to increase superficial circulation. It warms the area for further work, eases muscle spasm, stimulates the skin, passively stretches the muscles, relaxes the body (when performed at a slow pace) or prepares it for activity (fast pace), and feels structures underneath the skin in the muscle such as tight knots. It may be applied at a slow or fast rate. For the pre- and postperformance massages we will be using a kind of effleurage called smoothing,

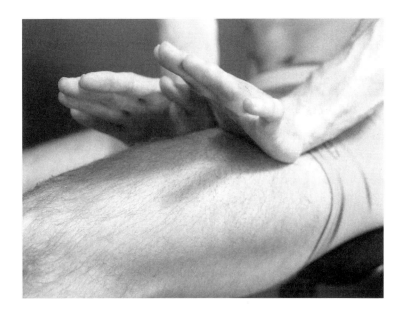

which is done without creme or oil. To familiarize yourself with the movement, try some smoothing on yourself: sit and place your palm of your hand
on your thigh, the quadriceps group of muscles. Now move the hand down
your thigh to the knee applying light pressure. Then move your hand back
up your thigh to your hip releasing the pressure on our leg, but still keeping
contact with the skin. When you release you'll still feel the light pressure
from just placing your hand on your leg. As you go down again, begin to
increase the pressure by leaning over with your body weight (this will help
the stroke get to deeper levels of the muscle).

This stroke works on the lymphatic and blood circulatory systems by
actually pushing them. With the friction from your hand and the hyper-
emia reflex, effleurage also starts to warm the muscle and tissues underneath the skin. When you put pressure on your skin, it stops the flow of
blood; as you release, the blood flows back in, causing the skin to appear
reddish and grow warm. Not only are nutrients moved in and metabolic
wastes such as lactic acid and other ions moved out of the superficial tissues, but the stroke's direction also helps the veins move the blood and
lymph back to the heart. (Note: the opposite direction is demonstrated in
my example above.)

In the extremities, effleurage should be done from the distal point (a relative point furthest from the heart) to the proximal point (a relative point closest to the heart): knee to hip, foot to knee, elbow to shoulder, and wrist to elbow. It can include more than one joint—the stroke can go from the foot to the hip or the wrist to the neck—depending on what is comfortable and feels good to the athlete. Executed with any part of the hand or forearm, effleurage starts and ends your massage. Throughout this book, we will refer to effleurage without creme as "smoothing."

Petrissage

Petrissage goes deeper than effleurage and is more specific to an area. Petrissage squeezes the blood out from deeper structures, relaxes muscle fibers, and warms the muscle fiber through body friction and from the

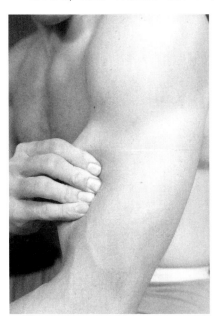

increased flow of blood. It is used to feel individual muscles or fibers, tendons, and ligaments. It loads the muscle with blood, milks the muscle of wastes and fatigue byproducts from overexertion. To get a feel for petrissage, grasp as much muscle as you can from the front of your upper arm (this is the biceps brachii and the brachialis) with the opposite hand. Lightly grasp and squish the muscle between your fingers and palm until the muscle warms and gets soft. Then you can apply greater pressure to work deeper into the muscle. You can do the same thing to a smaller area by just using your fingers and the thumb. This type of petrissage is called kneading. It is important to start as superficially as possible so the muscle will release and let you go

deeper. Otherwise the body will resist. These strokes are great for muscle bellies. Besides kneading, other forms of petrissage are grasping and lifting, which are often combined and are similar to kneading. The massager will grasp the tissue between the fingers and lift it away from the bone, jostle it (placing one or both hands on a muscle and then shake and move the tissue to loosen it up), roll it (moving your hands perpendicular or across the muscle), and broaden it (similar to rolling, but your other hand will go in the opposite direction to the first hand when moving across the muscle to spread or broaden the tissue).

The stroke goes into the tissue. It can be performed in any direction (usually parallel to the muscle you are working on). As with effleurage, it is important to end by going toward the heart. Petrissage is also effective treatment for muscle spasm, as it loosens the spasm to let the blood in. An example would be to knead the muscles on the back of the thigh (the hamstring group) up and down, but end by going up the hamstrings from the knee to the hip. Petrissage is great to use on soft structures, but is not good for massaging bony areas like the elbow or knee.

Compression

Compression is a form of petrissage that I will deal with separately here because of its special value and use in sports massage. To demonstrate compression, place the palm of your hand on the middle of your thigh while sitting down. Lean on your hand with your body weight. Then release the

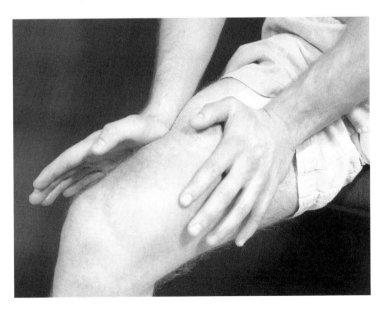

weight and repeat. This will create a pumping action. Keeping skin contact, move your hand gradually down your thigh as you pump. Compression strokes can also be done with a loose fist, the forearm, or even a foot (foot shiatsu). When doing compression make sure to squish (or compress) the muscle into the bone. Otherwise, you are just displacing the muscle but the fluids in the muscle are not being worked on. Think of squeezing out a wet sponge as opposed to merely pushing it around. The squishing gets more water out. Compression strokes are an excellent way for the massager to feel the tissues underneath the skin and at different levels: lighter pressure to feel superficial structures and more pressure to feel the deeper structures. The depth and speed of the stroke will determine what it will do to the athlete. Performing the stroke fast will invigorate and warm the tissue, while a slow pace will sedate, relax, and help pump the blood out.

Compression is great for muscle bellies, working large areas such as the adductors (inner thigh), assessing muscle tightness, and as a substitute for smoothing. Compression is not good for bony areas.

Trigger Point Work

Trigger point work is an excellent way to loosen chronic tight holding patterns in one's posture: tight lifted shoulders, crooked lower back, etc. Trigger points are areas of a muscle that are tight, sensitive, and painful. When pressure is applied to a trigger point, the accumulated pain will radiate out to other areas. You will know and understand when you hit a trigger point, because the athlete will indicate that the area is especially sensitive and painful. The athlete may holler, take a sharp, deep breath, or say "that's the spot that hurts!" Though trigger points are common, not everyone has one. They are unique to each person, but there are certain areas where they are most likely found. An example is the thumb trigger point, which can be found by pressing down into the meaty section below your thumb with the opposite thumb (while your hand is palm-up on the thigh), move around the area till you hit the most sensitive point, that is a trigger point (you may have more then one!). Start by using light pressure to find the trigger point, then increase the pressure to your pain threshold. Do not press in too deep and quickly, the muscle will let you in only if you are gentle. Otherwise it

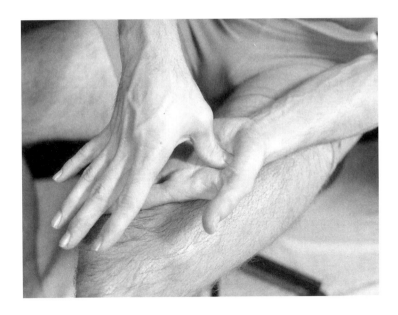

will feel as if the body part is being attacked and that will only increase the tightness.

Working the trigger point correctly will release tight muscle holding and break the pain cycle so the tissue can get blood and nutrients to heal and relax itself. A good analogy for a trigger point would be a kinked water hose. The pressure causes undue wear and tear on the hose. When the kink is worked out, there is a rush of fluid through the hose as the pressure is released. In the muscle, the kink is relieved by getting the needed extra nutrients to the tight tissues so that they are replenished and the pain and tension goes away. Trigger point work can relieve and loosen a tight muscle with very little other work to the muscle. The pressure should be applied to a specific area up to the pain threshold for an extended period of time (usually around 30 to 45 seconds) and then lightly and gently released. You may use a thumb, index finger with the middle finger bracing it—even an elbow can work nicely. Physiologically, the pressure will create increased blood flow after the pressure is let up. Since all you are doing is pressing and holding the pressure, the rate of stroke is the time you hold the pressure. The depth of the stroke should never go above an 8 or 9 on the 1–10 scale: a 1 is resting your palm on someone, and a 10 is the Dr. Spock death grip on *Star*

Trek. This stroke is used for muscle maintenance. Trigger point work is not for pre- and postevent massages because it is deep tissue work.

Friction

Another type of stroke used for deep tissue massage is friction. Friction can be done with the thumbs, fingers, or even the elbow. The pressure may be light for superficial areas or heavy to get the deeper areas. To familiarize yourself with the friction stroke, put your left arm on your leg with the palm down while sitting. Press the four right fingers into the muscles in the back of your forearm. Now move the fingers back and forth without sliding over 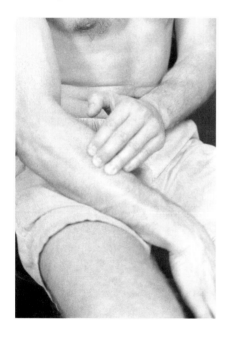 the skin. It is important to use the flat of a thumb or finger to press into the tissue, not the end part with the fingernail. The speed of the stroke through the skin may be fast for nonspecific, general friction, or slow for feeling tight areas and knots, specific friction.

Friction is used for increasing blood flow, finding and breaking up adhesions, stretching fibers, to feel and palpate specific tissues, and to be more specific than with any of the other strokes. It is used to loosen up scar tissue (but not keloid scars, which are red and raised) and to realign muscle fibers so that they will work freely. When the body's tissues work freely, the body uses less energy, the muscles pull more efficiently as they are supposed to, the tissues rub less against one another, which helps avoid overuse injuries such as tendinitis, tenosynovitis, and a slew of other avoidable injuries. The stroke brings in blood after placing pressure to a small area. The stroke can be circular for joint and bony areas, elongated with the muscle to stretch and lengthen tissues, or across the fibers to break apart bound tissues. Friction done to tight areas can be performed for 5 to 7 minutes continuously.

This stroke takes advantage of the colloidal properties (called thixotropy) of the tissues. Think of a hot butter knife melting down through a stick of butter—friction is one of the best, or most specific, ways to help the massager "see" what's going on in the body's deep tissue structures. It is important to pay attention to the client's facial expressions, body tenseness, references to pain, and other feedback in order to judge the effectiveness of how you are using the stroke. A beginner can get maximum benefits from friction by not trying to do too much, going too deep too fast, or by doing too many strokes. Doing too much can produce too much pain in the athlete so that they cannot relax, and insensitive overworking of a tightened area will aggravate the area and tighten it more. The experienced practitioner uses friction well to get the results he wants, while the athlete should enjoy the process of relaxing and releasing tightness.

Range of Motion

The next technique is range-of-motion (ROM) technique (look back to Exercise 1 in Chapter 2). ROM keeps and increases the joint's mobility through the entire movement range. These techniques free up adhered tissue, as well as warm the tissues and lubricate the joints. They also relax tight muscles, start to lubricate the joint capsule, tendons, muscles, bursa, and other tissues that rub over each other during movement, promote lymph and blood circulation, and increase limited range of motion. Each joint is made to move in certain planes of movement and in certain degrees of a circle. Try ROM technique by grabbing the end of your index finger with your other hand and straighten it so that it is fully extended, then bend at all the joints along the finger (just as if you were making a fist with one finger not all four).

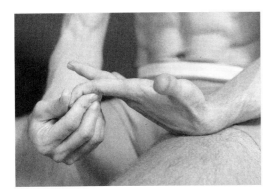 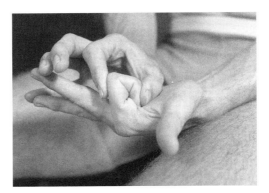

All the body's joints may be moved, but we will focus on the major ones: the ankle, knee, hip, neck, shoulder, elbow, and wrist. ROM techniques are used on the joints. Doing these techniques can be fun and may lead to new ways to loosen up the body. The movements are straight in one plane (lifting the leg up and down when you are on your back), circular (moving the shoulder joint in a wide circle like the backstroke), or a figure eight (a figure eight of the hip joint that can be larger or smaller at certain parts of the eight). The pace of the techniques may be slow, medium, or fast. The massager does the movement while the athlete stays relaxed. If you are doing this on your own, then you may be doing what is called active stretching (see below in stretching). This stroke is especially great for athletes because they need to have full range of motion in their joints in order to achieve their goals. The results that you get from range-of-motion techniques are similar to stretching, but it's the joint's movement that is important instead of the muscle stretch.

Stretching

Stretching is also used in sports massage because of its effectiveness and specificity. Stretching elongates fibers of muscle, tendon, and fascia. Stretching is great for loosening scar tissue and getting full range of motion back. It is important to warm up the tissue through light aerobic exercise before stretching to avoid tears and injury. A relevant analogy is two sticks, one in summer and one in winter. Because the stick in the summer is warmer and softer, it will bend and be flexible when stretched; the stick in winter will snap and break when stretched. Stretching involves putting the muscle and tendon at the greatest and tightest length that the muscle wants to handle— if the person goes too fast or too far it will signal the muscle to contract and hamper the stretch. Any stretch should be comfortable. There are many ways to stretch, but we will only use a few. They are static or holding stretches, active stretching, and PNF (proprioceptor neuromuscular facilitation) stretches.

In static stretching the massager holds the other person in one position in a way that keeps the muscle taut. The stretch is held in place for 10 to 60 seconds or longer so the tissue may relax and stretch further. The athlete should not hold his breath. The breath is natural and the person focuses the breath into the stretch to get a greater relaxation of the muscle.

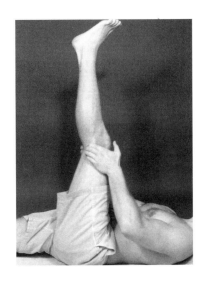

An active stretch is when the athlete moves the limb to be stretched in the opposite direction of the muscle's contraction. An example of an active hamstring stretch would be to keep the leg straight while lying on your back. Keep the leg straight as you contract the quads and hip flexors. Bring the leg straight up from the hip to its highest position, closest to 90 degrees. Remember to contract the quads not the hamstrings (the muscle being stretched). These active stretches are great for any pre-event massage or warm-up.

PNF stretches use the body's nervous system to help relax muscle tissue to get a deeper stretch. In one type of PNF stretch, the muscle is contracted against an immovable force, relaxed, and then statically stretched further to have a greater effect than just static stretching alone. To demonstrate this on yourself, place the back of your left hand on the left low back area. Grab the left elbow with your other hand and pull forward gently to stretch the back of the shoulder. The muscle you are stretching is called the infraspinatus. It is located on the back of the shoulder on the shoulder blade. Contract your elbow back without moving it (you can use between 10 and 90 percent of your maximum strength—50 percent is good). Hold the contraction for 8 seconds. Relax and release the tension after 8 seconds. Then pull your elbow further forward to stretch the shoulder again. Repeat these few steps 2 more times.

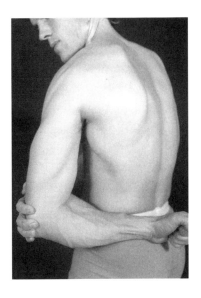

KEY POINTS:

1. Effleurage, which without oil or creme we will call smoothing, is a stroke over the skin. It is a transition or warming stroke. It can be a long or short stroke. It is used on the entire body. It affects the superficial circulation, relaxes the person, and lets them get used to your touch.

2. Petrissages are strokes that work deeper into the muscle tissue than effleurage. Some of the strokes are called kneading, grasping, lifting, jostling, rolling, and broadening. It is used to work the muscle bellies. It affects the deeper circulation, relaxes tight muscle tissue, and pumps the blood into and out of the muscle.

3. Compression is a form of petrissage. It is a pumping motion in and out of the tissue. It is also done on muscle bellies.

4. Trigger point work is holding constant pressure on an area of a muscle that is tight and painful. The pain will usually radiate to other areas of the body. The radiating pain is a key to finding a trigger point. The holding lasts at least 30 to 45 seconds. Trigger point work is done on muscle and musculo-tendon junctions. A milking of the point helps in relieving the pain and tightness.

5. Friction is a stroke that does not move over the skin. The stroke can go across (transverse), longitudinal, or in circular movements. The stroke is done on all parts of the body. It is used to break up adhesion or knots and to spread and realign tissue fibers.

6. Range-of-motion movements move a joint or joints through a full range of motions. The motion may go through the three planes. The movements relax tight muscles, lubricate and warm joints and tissue, and increase the range of motion.

7. Stretching is holding a body part so that a particular muscle or group of muscles is at its longest. Stretching should be held for at least 10 seconds and works very well between 30 seconds and 1 minute.

8. The depth and frequency of a stroke are interrelated. A deep stroke is long and slow. A superficial stroke is short and fast. The long and slow frequency will soothe and relax. A short and fast frequency will liven and energize.

EXERCISE

The purpose of this exercise is to practice all the strokes in this chapter on your thighs.

Start with smoothing. Go next to petrissage, compression, trigger point work, friction, range of motion, and stretching. Work the strokes on many different areas of the quads (by the hip, the outside of the knee, the inside of the knee, between the different muscle fibers, etc.).

Now use as many different body parts as you can to do the strokes. Use the heel of your hand for effleurage, the forearm for compression, the fist for friction, the elbow for trigger point work, and other combinations that you can think of.

Next do the strokes again. But this time, change the depth and frequency. Try the stroke faster. Try the strokes slower. Try making the strokes longer over the body. Try making the strokes shorter. How does the stroke's components change how the stroke feels on your body?

Practice these exercises on other parts of your body. How do they work for the calves, the neck, the hands, the shoulder, the butt? Experiment.

1: Start with your partner lying on her stomach. Her head is turned to the right side. Her arms are in a comfortable position.

2: Move to her right side of her back.

3: Place the heel of your hands onto the muscles next to the left side of the spine. You are reaching across her spine.

4: Press with compression strokes as light as you can by just leaning your weight onto the body. Do not try to go deep into the muscle or try to go fast.

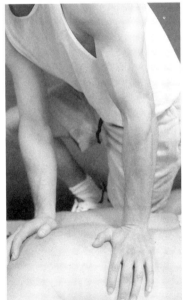

5: Move over the entire back by changing sides if you feel like it. Work the back of the legs, front of the legs, chest, and arms. Take about 15 minutes to cover the entire body.

6: After you are done, feel how your body feels: tight, loose, energized, or tired. Ask the person you worked on how they feel: are they relaxed, energized, tight. Do they feel that you got deeper than you thought you worked?

If you do not have a partner, get on all fours to crawl. Crawl around the room as slowly as you can. Release the weight in your arms and legs as lightly as possible as you move them. Place the arms and legs back onto the ground as softly as you can. Do this for 10 minutes. Make sure to breathe deeply and slowly. Try to breathe down into your belly. Afterward, ask your self how you feel emotionally and physically. Scan your attention over your entire body to see if areas are tight, painful, loose, or energized. Did they get that way from the exercise or from how you held yourself previously?

Pre-Event Self Sports Massage

A pre-event self sports massage routine will be given in this chapter. Each sport will have special areas of emphasis to be given later in the chapter (pp. 57–75). It is important to have the athlete's goals in mind: to warm and stretch the athlete. One way you can use these routines is to memorize them and then do them on yourself. Another way is to read the routine into a tape recorder and then play it back as you do the massage. If you do talk into a recorder, remember to leave yourself enough time between paragraphs to do the massages. Do not forget to warm up lightly before these massages.

Quadriceps and Adductors

1. Sit on the ground with your right leg straight and your left leg bent, with the bottom of the left foot by the right knee.

2. Place your hands on the right quads and smooth the leg at a fast to vigorous pace for 20 seconds.

3. Place the palms of your hands above the knee and sink your weight into the muscles. With your weight in the muscle, massage with your hands in a circular pattern as you work the muscles. The hands may move together as a unit or out of phase, opposite each other. The hands may move clockwise or counterclockwise at a medium pace. Move up and down the

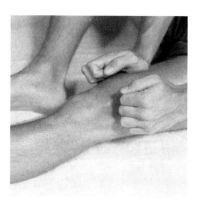

thigh from the knee to the hip. Move from the inside (groin, adductor area of the thigh) to the outside of the thigh as you massage for 30 seconds. Get the area from the hip to the knee joint.

4. Compress down into the thigh with the palm of your hands. Move up and down from the hip to just above the back of the knee. Then move from the front of the thigh to the back of the thigh. Move up the thigh as you do this till you get to the hip.

5. Smooth the leg at a medium to fast pace from the knee to the hip for 10 seconds with the palm of your hands. It is easier to do this by leaning the upper body back. This will use the body weight and not the shoulder muscles.

6. Finish by shaking the area: place the palm of your hand on the muscle and shake it at a fast pace for at least 10 seconds.

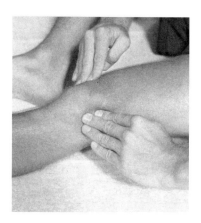

Knee

1. Stay in the same seated position as above.

2. Place the tips of your fingers around the kneecap.

3. Apply circular friction around the kneecap and knee joint area for 10 seconds. It is important to do the top and bottom of the kneecap. This is where the tendons attach.

4. Smooth around the front and back of the knee joint for 10 seconds.

Lower Leg

1. Stay in the seated position.
2. Bend the straightened leg, the knee is pointing up to the ceiling, and the foot is on the ground.
3. Place the palms of your hands just above the ankle and smooth the area up from the ankle to the knee for at least 10 seconds.
4. Place one of your palms on the bone on the inside part (the right hand for the left leg and the left hand for the right leg) of your lower leg and the other on the muscles on the outside of the leg. The outside hand will be doing the most movement because it is working the muscles. Do circular movements up and down the leg between the knee and the ankle. This is the shinsplint area. Do not do anything too painful. Do for at least 10 seconds.
5. Compress the muscles by interlocking your fingers and squeezing into the bone and outside muscle.
6. Smooth the area of the lower leg for at least 10 seconds.
7. Finish by shaking the muscles with the palms of your hands for at least 10 seconds.

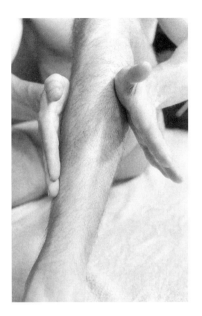

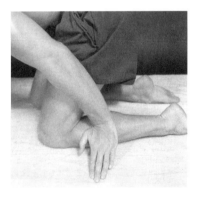

Calves

1. Move your body onto all fours. You will be leaning back on the legs more than the arms.
2. Place one hand on the corresponding calf (right on right or left on left), and compress

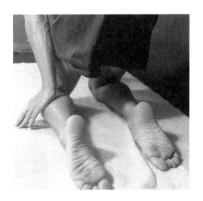

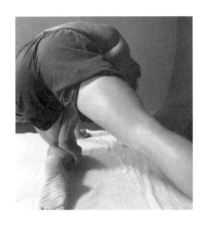

down into the outside of the calf. Start light with a medium speed and slow the speed as you go deeper. Compress down and up the leg.

3. Shake the muscles worked on.

4. Return to all fours.

5. Straighten the opposite leg out at a 45-degree angle away from the body, and place corresponding hand onto the inside of the calf.

6. Compress the inside of the calves from the knee to the ankle at a medium speed and depth for at least 10 seconds.

Foot

1. Stay on all fours with one leg out at a 45-degree angle.

2. Place the opposite hand's palm or fist (left on right, right on left) on the sole of the foot to compress the muscles on the bottom of the foot. Massage for at least 10 seconds.

3. Stop by the heel of the foot and, with constant pressure applied with the fist, press into the bottom of the foot and slide down the foot to the toes.

4. Move to a seated position with the right leg just about straightened and the knee to the outside.

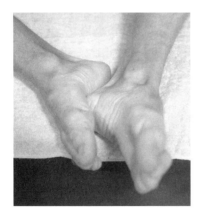

5. Press the left heel into the arch of the right foot. Use the left heel to do circular compressions to the right foot. Bring the foot you are working on closer to you with the knee out to the side.

6. Smooth the bottom of the foot with the heel of the opposite hand.

Hamstrings

1. Lie down flat on your back. The left leg is flat on the floor. The right leg is bent and lifted to the chest.

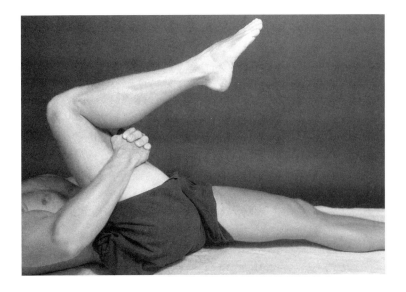

2. Interlace the fingers and smooth the right hamstrings from the knee to the hip with the heel of both hands.

3. Return to the area around the knee and squeeze the hamstrings between the heels of your interlaced hands at a medium pace. Squeeze this area between the knee and the hip.

4. Make your right hand into a fist. Place the left hand over on top of the right hand. Compress the fist into the hamstrings from the knee to the hip in straight lines.

5. Switch hands so the left hand becomes a fist as you get to the inside of the hamstrings.

6. Smooth with both hands then finish by shaking the muscle area.

Repeat with the legs reversed for work on the left side.

STRETCHES
Hamstrings

1. Lie flat on your back.
2. Raise the right leg. The left foot is flat on the floor.
3. Place your hands behind the right leg below the knee with your fingers interlaced.

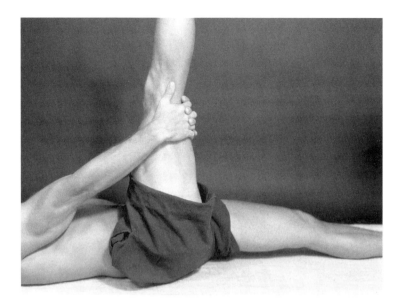

4. Pull gently with your arms and bring the leg closer to your chest till you feel a stretch. Keep the leg straight. Hold for 20–30 seconds.

5. Repeat on same leg if desired or do the stretch on the other side.

6. To do an activated isolated stretch, contract the quads as you raise the leg to stretch the hamstrings.

7. Hold the leg at the end range of motion to stretch for up to 10 seconds.

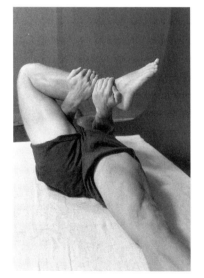

8. Release and lower the leg slowly to the floor.

9. Repeat the contraction and raising of the leg 3–5 times. As you do this, think of relaxing the hamstrings as you contract the quads. Remember to breathe.

Piriformis

1. Lie flat on your back.

2. The left leg is flat on the floor. Take the right leg by the ankle and place it on the left leg across the knee. The right foot is on the left side of the left leg by the knee and the rest of the right leg is on the right side.

3. The right knee falls to the outside of the right side.
4. Place both your hands with fingers interlaced behind the left knee. The right forearm by the elbow is on the inner thigh of the right leg, pressing it away.
5. Raise the left leg to your chest and feel the stretch in your right butt. To get a deeper stretch, press the leg away with the elbow and pull the legs closer to the chest. Hold for 20–30 seconds.
6. Repeat 2–3 more times if desired, then repeat on the other side.

Iliotibial Band

1. Lie on your back, with both your knees bent. The feet are flat on the floor.
2. Place the right leg across the left leg as if you were crossing your legs. The left foot is on the ground and the right foot is in the air.
3. Drop the crossed legs to the left side (away from the leg to be stretched). Hold for 20–30 seconds.
4. Repeat 2–3 times, then repeat on the other side.

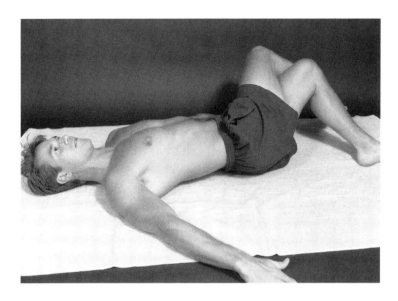

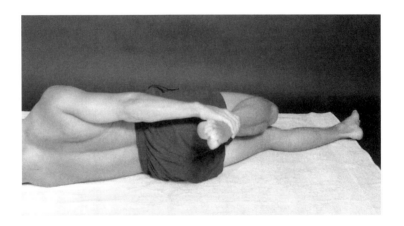

Quadriceps

1. Roll on your left side and bend the right leg so the right foot is near the right butt cheek.
2. Raise the left arm straight above the head and rest your head on the upper arm area.
3. Grab the right foot at the ankle area and pull the leg back to your back. Be careful to tighten the abdominals to let the leg stretch. Do not just arch your back, feel the stretch. Hold for 20–30 seconds.
4. Repeat 2–3 times, then repeat on the other side.

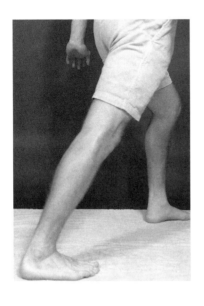

Calves

1. Stand up by a wall or step.
2. Place the right foot on the step so the toes are raised and the heel is on the floor. Feel the stretch in the calves. Hold the stretch for 20–30 seconds.
3. Repeat 2–3 times, or repeat on the other side.
4. Another way to stretch the calves is to use a wall. Place the right leg behind you.
5. The left leg is bent in front of the right leg.
6. The hands are on a wall or the floor in

front of you. If on the floor the body is bent at the waist in a V shape.

7. Lean forward to feel the stretch in the right leg.

Soleus

1. Lie on your back.
2. Raise the right knee onto your chest with the leg bent at the knee.
3. Grab your right foot by the toes and front of the foot with both hands.
4. Press the heel of the right foot away from the body. The muscle that is stretched is underneath the calf muscle and closer to the ankle. Hold for 20–30 seconds.
5. Repeat 2–3 times, then repeat on the other side.

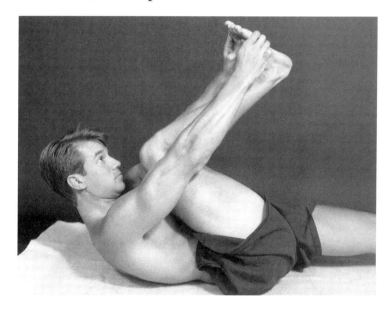

Tibialis Anterior

1. Sit on both knees with the feet behind and underneath the butt. The upper body weight is on the heels of the feet.
2. Lean forward slightly and grab the left foot by the toes. The hands are on either side of the front of the foot.

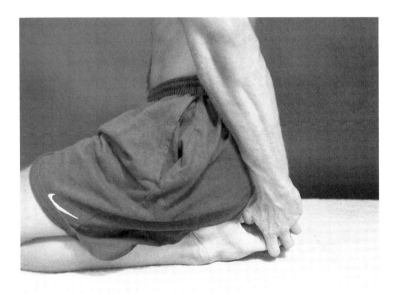

3. Lean your weight onto the heels and feel the stretch in the front of the left lower leg. Hold for 20–30 seconds.

4. Repeat 2–3 times, then repeat on the other side.

Groin

1. Lie on your back with your legs straight at the knee and your feet on the floor.

2. Drop your right knee to the right side toward the floor.

3. Place your right hand on the inside right knee and push down to the floor.

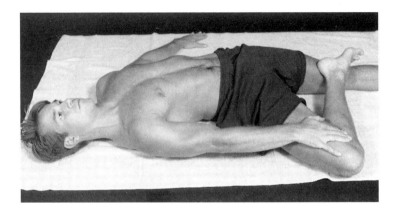

4. Lean the body and left knee slightly to the left side with the rest of your body. Hold for 20–30 seconds.
5. Repeat 2–3 times, or repeat on the other side.

UPPER BODY

The massages can be done lying down, sitting, or standing up.

Chest

1. Lie on your back. Legs can be bent or straight.
2. Press the fingers of your right hand on your left pectoral muscle.
3. Smooth the muscle from breastbone to shoulder. Get the bottom, middle, and top of the chest.
4. Press into the chest with the heel of your hand and do some circular compressions (compress the tissue and move the hand in circular motions in the tissue) to the entire pectoral muscle. Massage at a medium pace and depth.
5. Finish the area by smoothing with the right hand.
6. Repeat on the other side.

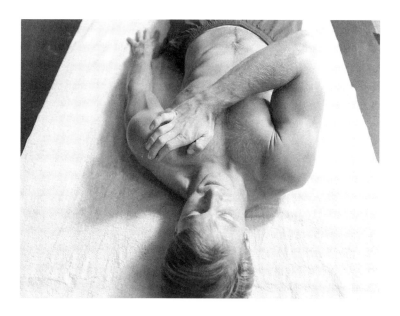

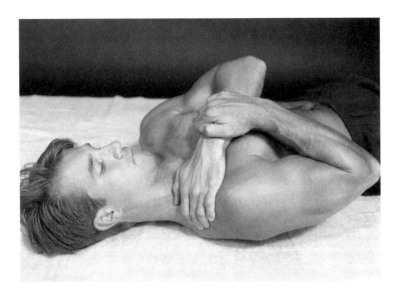

Upper Traps

1. Lie on your back. The legs can be bent or straight.
2. Grab the muscle on the upper back between the neck and the right shoulder with the opposite (left) hand.
3. With your right hand, grab the left arm around the elbow. You will be using the right arm to get more massage pressure.
4. Knead the muscle (grab and release the tissue between the finger and heel of the hand) from the neck to the shoulder at least 3 times. Start with light pressure at a medium pace. Increase the pressure at the same pace (medium) as the muscle warms and loosens.
5. Next, cup your left hand so the fingers are held together.
6. Press the pads of the fingertips into the muscle.
7. Circular friction with the fingers between the shoulder blade, neck, and the shoulder at a medium speed.
8. Finish by smoothing the area massaged.
9. Repeat on the other side.

Upper Arm

The deltoid, triceps, and biceps are massaged in this section.

1. Grab the right outside shoulder with your left hand.

2. Knead the muscle (deltoid) from the outside edge of the chest around back to the outside of the shoulder blade 3 times. Start with light pressure and increase to medium pressure as the tissue warms. Go at a medium to fast pace.

3. Knead down the front of the upper arm (biceps muscle) to the elbow and around the outside to the back of the arm (triceps muscle).

4. Knead up the triceps to the back of the deltoid and around again at least 3 times.

5. Finish the area massaged by smoothing or shaking the whole area vigorously.

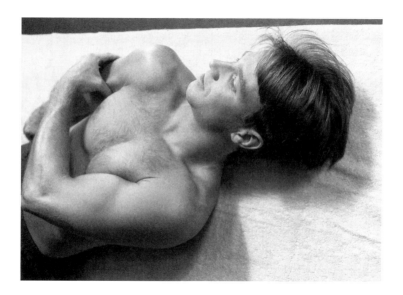

Forearm
1. Take a deep breath in.
2. Breathe out as you sit up. Legs are straight.
3. Place your right forearm on your right leg with the palm down.
4. Compress the muscles on the top of the forearm with the palm of your left hand. Compress down from the elbow to the wrist at least 3 times at a medium to fast pace.
5. Cup your left hand with the fingers together.
6. Press the pads of your fingertips in at the top of the wrist by the elbow.
7. Circular friction the wrist extensors (the top or back of the forearm

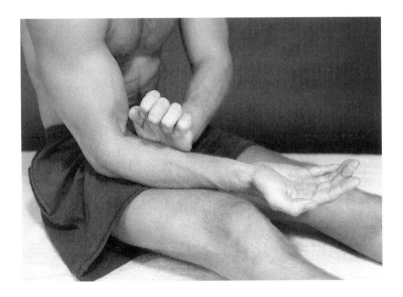

muscles that you are working on) down from the elbow to the wrist. Do 3 times at a light pace and depth.

8. Turn the right arm so that the palm is now up.

9. Compress the wrist flexors (the inside forearm muscles) with the palm of your left hand from your elbow to the wrist. Compress the whole inside forearm from inside to the outside as well as top to bottom at a medium pace at least 3 times. Start with light pressure.

10. Friction the inside forearm like Step 7.

11. Repeat the strokes on other side.

Hand

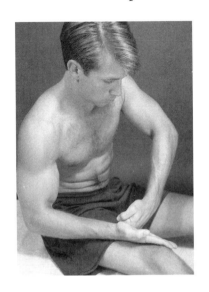

1. Sit in the same position as above.

2. The right hand is on the leg and the palm is up.

3. Make a fist with the left hand and do compression with the knuckles of the fist into the palm of your other hand. Get the muscles of the thumb and the little finger. The muscles are located on the inside and outside of the palm. Compress at a light pressure and pace at least 3 times.

4. Grab the left hand in your right hand so the fingers are on the back of the left hand and the palm and the right hand is pressing the muscles at the base of the thumb.

5. Spread the palm of the left hand out with the right hand by pressing the right palm into the left hand muscles. Do this at least 3 times at a medium to fast pace.

6. Turn your left hand over so the palm is down and grab the little finger side of your left palm with the right hand's fingers.

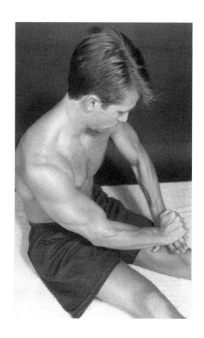

7. Place the right palm on the back of the left hand.

8. Spread the outside of the left hand by applying pressure with the right fingers to the muscles at the base of the left little finger. Do 3 times at a light pressure and medium pace.

9. Grab each of the left hand fingers with your right hand and slowly do range-of-motion techniques.

10. Repeat on the other side.

11. After you massage both sides, rub the palms of your hands together vigorously.

Trunk

1. Stand up with your legs about shoulder-width apart and your knees slightly bent.

2. Place both palms of your hands on your stomach, in the middle of your body just below your ribs.

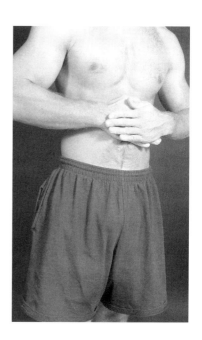

3. Slowly circle your hands to the left side, down to the left hip, over to the right hip, up to the right ribs, and back to the left as you rub your abdomen. Do 3 times.

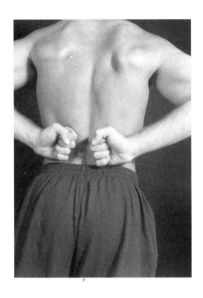

4. Twist your upper body slightly to the same side you are on. Twist to the left as you go to the left and twist to the right as you are at the bottom of the circle and going to the right. Repeat this circle at least 5 times. Only go in this clockwise direction because this is how your large intestines run: up on the right, across the top, and down the left. Doing the smoothing also helps in aiding digestion and bowel movements.

5. Stop and place the palms of your hands on the corresponding sides (left to left and right to right) of your lower back.

6. Rub or smooth the area from your hips to ribs at least 5 times. Go at a medium pace and depth.

7. Make your hand into fists and place the backs of your hands on the same side of the low back area.

8. Press your knuckles into the muscles on either side of your spine.

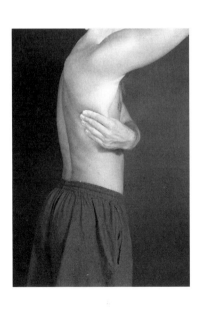

9. Lightly friction across these muscles with 1-inch strokes going from the spine out. Friction the area from your hipbone up to the back of the ribs, out from the spine to your sides. Friction this area for 1 minute.

10. Place your left palm on the right side of your body by the hip.

11. Smooth the area from your hip up to your armpit and back down at least 5 times at a light depth and medium pace.

12. Stop and now grab the outside right back muscles with the left hand up by the armpit but further back to the shoulder

blade. Knead the muscles from the right scapula to the hip at least 5 times.

13. Repeat on the other side.

Butt

1. Separate your legs a little further than shoulder-width apart.

2. Grab each side of your butt with the corresponding hand (left on left and right on right).

3. Knead the muscles all around your butt between the fingers and the palms of your hands. These are dense tissues so really get in there and loosen them up. Knead for at least 30 seconds. Start with light pressure and medium pace.

Finish the area by patting all around the gluts.

STRETCHES

Infraspinatus

1. Stand and place the left arm straight across the body at nipple or armpit height.

2. With the right arm, hook the left arm above the elbow with the right front elbow region. The left arm is now locked into the right arm.

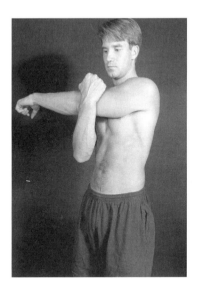

3. Pull the left arm away but toward the right side using the right arm. Feel the stretch behind the shoulder on the outside of the left shoulder blade. Hold the stretch for at least 10 seconds

4. Repeat if necessary, and then repeat on the other side.

Triceps

1. Reach and place the left hand on the top of the left shoulder.

2. Place the right hand on the left elbow.

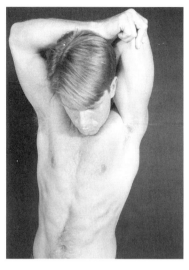

3. Push the left arm up to the ceiling while keeping the left hand in contact with the shoulder. Do not arch the back.
4. Tighten the abdominals.
5. Hold the stretch at the highest point or at the deepest stretch for at least 10 seconds.
6. Repeat the stretch if necessary and then repeat on the other side.

Traps and Infraspinatus

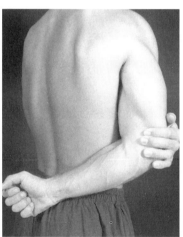

1. Place the back of the right hand on the same side of the lower back. The right elbow is out to the side.
2. Reach across the body with the left arm and grab the right elbow.
3. Pull the elbow to the opposite (left) side. Make sure that the shoulders do not rise up. To increase the stretch, drop the head to the side that the arm is being pulled to: for a right side stretch, the left arm is pulling the right arm to the left side and the head drops to the left. Hold the stretch for at least 10 seconds.
4. Repeat the stretch if necessary, and then repeat the sequence on the other side.

Lats

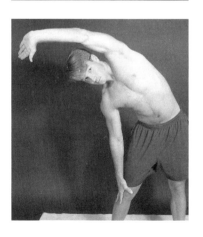

1. Keep standing with the feet past shoulder width for support.
2. Lean to right as you raise the left arm over your head and to the right. Feel the stretch on the outside of the back. Hold for at least 10 seconds.
3. Repeat the stretch if necessary, then do the other side.

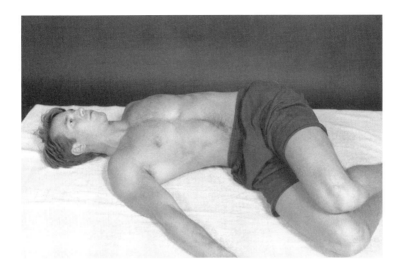

Low Back

1. Lie on your back with your arms out to the sides. The legs are bent at the knees. The knees are straight up in the air.
2. Drop the knees to the right side so the body twists. The knees are by or on the ground. Try to keep your upper back flat on the ground. Hold the stretch for at least 10 seconds.
3. Repeat the stretch, then repeat again on the other side.

SPORTS-SPECIFIC MASSAGE TIPS

Running, Hiking, Jogging

In any type of running, hiking, or jogging event—the hurdles, sprints, marathons, or jogging—the massager will spend most of the time on the legs, butt, abs, and lower back. The massager will also stretch the same areas: legs, butt, and trunk (all around the midsection). If the event is high intensity running or hiking, as in sprinting, hurdles, or heavy backpacking, the massager will massage and stretch the shoulder, chest, and upper back. The massager does ankle range of motions: circle the ankle in the largest circles, point the toes up and down, turn ankle in and out, and squeeze the toes in and spread them out. The athlete can do circular compressions, smoothing, or shaking and jostling to the abs, low back, butt, quads, hamstrings, calves, and front lower leg.

Runners, hikers, and joggers must worry about overuse injuries, pulled muscles, and falling injuries. These injuries could include shinsplints, blisters, pulled or strained hamstrings, and sprained ankles or wrists. When falling, the athlete must worry about cuts and bruises, not to mention the elements of weather—hot, cold, wet, snowy, etc., type of combination weather—and dogs and other animals that could hurt them. These athletes should do lunge stretches, groin stretches, calf and soleus stretches, ankle and hip range of motions, and smoothing and shaking the body from below the ribs.

The lunge stretch:

1. Stand up straight with the arms relaxed.
2. Step forward with one leg straight in front of that hip (not to the other side or the outside).
3. Stand with one leg in front and bent at the knee and hip, and the back leg bent at the hip, knee, and ankle to the back.
4. Complete the groin stretch by bringing the legs out to the sides as far as possible. Hands are on the ground for balance and support. One gets up from this position by moving the toes then the heels in slightly and bending at the back.

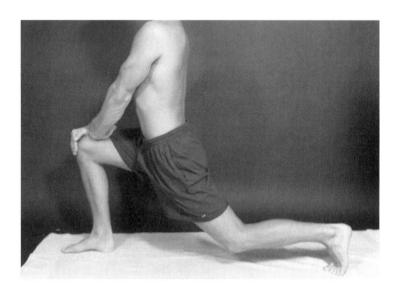

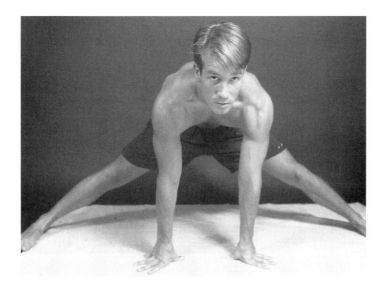

The calf stretch is described above (see illustration on page 46). The soleus stretch is the same, but the knee of the stretched leg is bent to get the muscle underneath (see illustration on page 47). The range of motions of the hip are raising the knee up to the chest and back down to the ground as the athlete is on her back.

Tennis and Racquetball

The massager will spend most of his time on the shoulder, forearms, adductors, hamstrings, and calves. He will also stretch these areas. The massager can do circular compressions, smoothing, and shaking and jostling to the legs, trunk, and shoulders before a match or practice. The athlete does wrist and ankle rotations or shakes to warm up these vital areas.

A tennis or racquetball player must be aware of overuse injuries, falling injuries, and one-sidedness injuries (most tennis or racquetball players only use one hit and serve arm and favor the forehand or backhand). The overuse injuries happen to the shoulders, forearm extensors by the elbow (tennis elbow), and wrist. The falling injuries happen to the ankle or groin and the one-sidedness injuries happen to the shoulder, elbow, wrist, and low back. These athletes must also be careful of being hit by the flying projectiles.

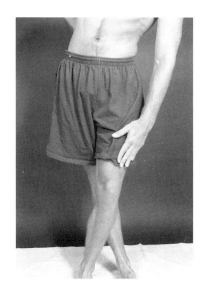

Great stretches for these athletes are the lunge and groin stretch shown in running.

Another great stretch is the standing iliotibial stretch:

1. Stand with legs shoulder-width apart and arms at the sides.

2. Plant the left leg on the ground and step in front with the right leg and to the side of the left foot with the right foot.

<u>3.</u> Then lean the body weight to the left side and stretch the upper body to the right to make a slight V in the body. The stretch is felt in the left outside leg and runs down the leg to at least the knee. Hold this stretch for at least 10 seconds and preferably longer to stretch this fascia.

4. You can also knead the shoulders with your hands. Other great areas to massage are the lower back, trunk (twisting stretches), shoulder range of motions, and wrist shaking.

Baseball

A baseball player uses his shoulders, upper arms, wrist, legs, and trunk when playing baseball. He needs these areas to work correctly to transfer the forces produced by the legs to work on the ball or bat. Baseball players must be careful of injuries to the elbow, forearm, wrist, shoulder, low back, and the hamstrings. All these injuries can happen from a collision with someone or the ground, or overuse by the repetitiveness of the sport (most baseball players only use one arm to throw, bat from one side, and sit behind a plate for over 3 hours).

The athletes should get the neck, traps, shoulder, upper arm, elbow, forearm, wrist, and hand massage. The lower back and hamstrings should also be emphasized. A pitcher will stretch out the arm. The triceps stretch is described above in the general workout. This stretch works the front of the shoulder and the chest muscles:

1. Bring both arms to the back and clasp the hands.

2. Raise the arms to the back and up. Hold the stretch at its highest point for at least 10 seconds, release, and repeat.

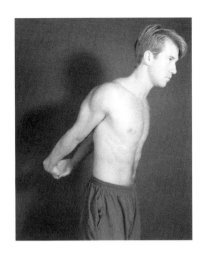

Then do the infraspinatus stretches described above in the general workout. To stretch the subscapularis muscle:

1. Stand up with the legs shoulder-width apart and the arms at the sides. The elbow of the right arm is bent to a 90-degree angle.

2. The right hand grasps an immovable object like a tree or the corner of a wall.

3. Then turn away from the hand on the wall while keeping the elbow at the side. Hold the stretch for at least 10 seconds and then repeat.

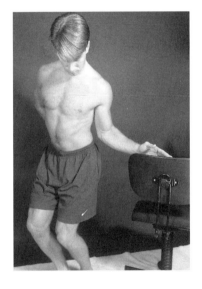

A catcher will also stretch out his quads, hamstrings, and lower back.

The first basemen will stretch the arms and legs with particular attention to the hamstrings and groin to increase the stretch to catch the ball thrown to first base. The side that a baseball player uses will get the most attention in stretching and massage, but, as any athlete should train and massage, the other side must also get worked. Another great stretch for baseball players is the press-up.

1. Lie down on your stomach with hands underneath the chest.

2. Press the upper body up, keeping the legs and hips on the floor.

3. Then look up to complete the stretch of the abdominals and front of the neck. Hold the stretch for at least 10 seconds and repeat.

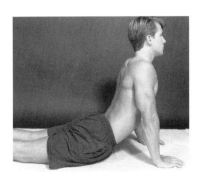

Basketball

A basketball player uses the entire body when she jumps, shoots, passes, twists when rebounding, and sprints when running the floor. The basketball player must get the entire body warmed and stretch out to play this game. The basketball player must contend with injuries to the ankles, shins, lower back, overuse injuries to the legs, jammed fingers, elbows to the head, and contusions from body contact.

The athlete will work the lower back, quads, hamstrings, calves, groin, feet, shoulder, and forearms. Basketball players need to spend more time in a stretch and massaging the area that is stretched because of the large number of games that they play. In one lower back and hamstrings stretch:

1. Lie on the your back.
2. Bring the right knee to the chest. The right knee is bent. The stretch is in the hamstrings and the lower back (see illustration on page 43).
3. Hold the stretch and knead the hamstrings with both hands. The kneading may be done on any stretch to the lower body and any stretch to one side of the upper body.

Two other great stretches for basketball are for the shoulders.
1. On your knees facing a wall, place both hands on the wall in front, and keep the hands there.
2. Lower the upper body. This stretches the lats, chest, and lower part of the shoulder capsule.

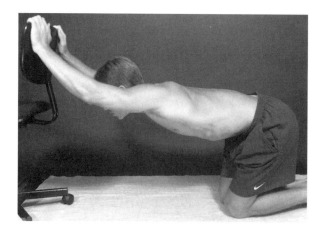

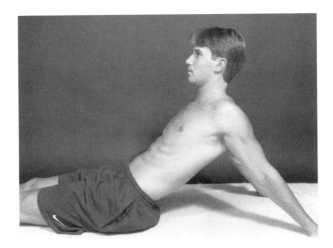

For the second stretch:

1. Sit on the ground with your legs out straight.

2. Place your arms behind your body.

3. Move the body forward to stretch the chest and shoulder.

Bicycling

Road and mountain bikers are athletes who go long distances and ride for a very long time. These athletes must worry about overuse injuries and falling injuries. These athletes must "sit" for long periods and thus the hamstrings and low back may be tight and cause low back pain. Bikers also get shin-splints from the toe clips, shoes, and the long period of using the ankle in only one way. Bikers also fall because of the terrain, other bikers, fatigue, or technical problems. The injuries caused by falling are to the skin of the legs, arms, and hands, shoulder and upper arm injuries from hitting the ground, and head injuries (always wear a helmet).

The areas that bikers will massage and stretch are the thighs (quads and hamstrings), hips, lower leg (front and back), low back, shoulder, arms, wrists, and neck.

One stretch is great for the soleus muscle, hips, and low back:

1. Stand with the feet a little wider than shoulder-width apart and the arms at your side.

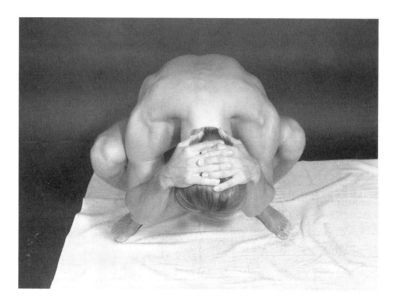

2. Squat down so the butt is below the knees, upper body by the knees.

3. Put the hands behind the head and pull chin to chest.

4. Hold the stretch for at least 10 seconds and then repeat.

Another stretch for a biker is the lunge stretch. This stretch is shown in the running section (see illustration on page 58). The range-of-motion technique "bookcases" is as follows:

1. Lie down on the ground on your back. The knees are bent and in the air, feet are on the ground.

2. Drop the right knee to the right side and hold for a few seconds.

3. Drop the left knee to the right and twist the body to the right.

4. Hold this position for a few seconds, raise the left leg to the beginning position, then raise the right to the beginning position.

5. Then drop the left knee to the left side, hold, and drop the right knee to the left side. The knees are brought back up one at a time to the starting position. The dropping of the knees is repeated at least 5 times. Synchronize the breaths so you breathe out as the knee is dropped, and breathe in on the holding, between positions.

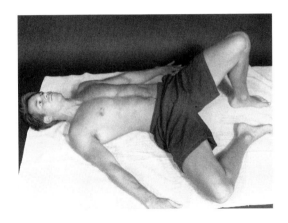 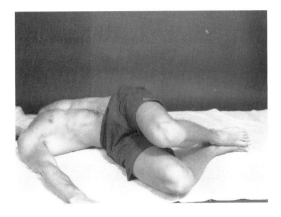

One important massage stroke for bikers is to jostle, tapot, knead, compress, shake, or smooth the quads and hamstrings vigorously before the race.

Bowling

Bowlers try to throw a heavy round object the same way 10 to 21 times a game. In bowling, the body twists, bends, and throws. The bowler usually only uses one arm to throw this heavy ball down the lane. The way the body bends and twists along with the heaviness of the ball and the repetitiveness of the action can help cause a trauma to the body. The low back, shoulder, hips, hamstrings, back, forearm, and wrist are all important areas.

The athlete must stretch and warm the torso. Bowling is a sport and one must prepare for bowling as such. Proper cardiovascular warm-up before pre-event sports massage is imperative. It will help the massage and stretches, help you avoid injuries, burn calories, and help your game. Here is a stretch for the abdominals.

1. Sit on a chair, arms at your side on your hips.
2. Lean the upper body back and look up.
3. Take in a deep breath, push the stomach out, hold the breath, and breathe out slowly, leaning forward to the starting position. The breathing out should take over 10 seconds and it helps to do this by breathing out the mouth.

The next stretch is for the lower back.

1. Stand up with the feet shoulder-width apart and the arms at your sides.

2. Breathe out and lean to the right side.

3. Reach over the body with the left arm to increase the stretch and to help stretch the lats (see bottom illustration on page 56).

4. Hold the stretch for at least 10 seconds, take a deep breath in, and return to the starting position.

5. Repeat on the other side and then get both sides again. The hamstrings and hips should also be stretched.

A massage stroke that the athlete can do for the torso is:

1. Stand, feet shoulder-width apart and arms at your sides.

2. Turn the upper body to the right, reach over with a cupped left hand as far back as possible to the midsection, and press the fingers into the lower back.

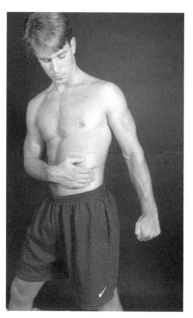

3. Turn to the left and smooth the right side of the abdominals with the left hand. Repeat the turning and stroke on the same side at least 3 times and then massage the other side.

The bowler can also, jostle, knead, compress, tapot, smooth, or shake the arm being used to bowl the bowling ball, the low back, and legs.

Dance and Aerobics

A dancer uses her whole body. She twists, jumps, stands on her toes, holds other dancers in the air, and every other type of combination of body movements that a choreographer can think up. These athletes must really do massage, as most of them do now. They get overuse injuries and trauma from the extremeness of the movements. The whole body is worked on, and the emphasis of the pre-event sports massage will depend on the particular dance that will be done. What are the major areas that could get injured? These are the areas to massage: the entire body from the neck down—neck, shoulders, back, low back, hips, abdominals, quads, hamstrings, groin, calves, shins, and feet.

For stretches, dancers should hold the stretches for a long time: 1–5 minutes. A dancer usually has a routine of stretches that they have practiced since the day they started. In addition to stretches, add circular compressions, jostling, shaking, and smoothing to the muscle that is being stretched before and after the stretch.

Golf

Golf is a sport of (hopefully) long walks between a smooth, clean stroke. Unfortunately, these clean and effortless strokes don't always happen. Golf is a sport that must be done for a long period of time to master it. The games are long (9, 18, 36 holes) and in warm to hot sunny weather. Golfers get overuse and trauma injuries. A golfer must also watch out for dehydration and other weather injuries (overheating in the summer; frostbite in the winter, fall, and spring; lightning, and rain). Some major golf injuries are golf elbow (overuse or trauma to the inside forearm muscles), low back pain, and pulled muscles (hamstring, shoulder, arm, back). A golfer uses a dominant side more than the other side. So one side may be more developed than the other. The stroke entails the whole body to work in unison so the ball will travel on its desired trajectory. A golfer will massage and stretch the lower back, trunk, hips, shoulders, and inside of the forearm to get the wrist muscles.

Great stretches for golfers are the lunge stretch (shown in running—see illustration on page 58), the "bookcase" (in bowling—see illustration on page 65), and the following one for the lower back:

1. Lie on your back, legs out straight and arms at your side.
2. Bend the right leg at the hip and knee so the knee is pointing straight up.
3. Lower the right knee to the left side so the right leg goes on top of the

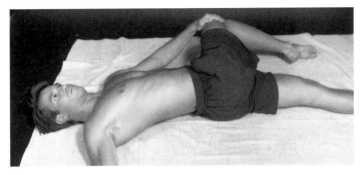

left leg. The back will now rise off the ground, but try to keep it flat. Hold the stretch for at least 10 seconds and then return to the starting position and repeat on the other side.

4. Another way to do this stretch is to keep the right leg straight as you bring the right leg to the ground. The leg may not make it to the ground or you will have to lower the leg so the foot stays closer to the left foot.

This stretch also gets the lower back and the iliotibial band on the outside of the leg. The iliotibial band can be stretched while standing up (shown in the tennis and racquetball section—see illustration on page 60). The infraspinatus stretch, another great one, is shown in the general workout (see illustration on page 55).

A golfer will massage the areas that he must be careful not to injure: forearm, wrist, shoulder, and low back. Smoothing, swinging the arms in circles (a range-of-motion technique), and twisting the body are all great to do before each stroke.

Football

Football is a collision sport. It is fast. The athletes are fast and heavy. This mix makes for a ferocious sport. A football player must be in top shape to play this game. The athlete must also be able to survive the progressively colder season with the minimum of injuries. This makes the week between games extremely important for the athlete and team. The athletes must heal, practice, and prepare for the next opponents. Football players can have just about any injury. They can break bones, tear muscles, have sprains, strains, bruises, scrapes, cuts, concussions, and more. The massager must deal with the soft-tissue injuries. The areas that need attention are the neck, shoulders, back, low back, quads, hamstrings, and ankles.

The massager will pay attention to the athlete's particular position when doing the pre-event sports massage. The position of the player and the role of the player will affect the massage. A quarterback will massage shoulders, arms, trunk, and low back. A running back will massage and stretch his legs, low back, shoulders, and forearms. Linemen will massage and stretch the legs, back, low back, trunk, and shoulders. Receivers and defensive backs massage and stretch their legs, back, low back, and shoulders.

Neck movements and rolls are done with the athlete standing or sitting on a chair.

1. Start by nodding "yes."
2. Drop the chin to the chest and then look up. Do this movement at least 5 times and then come back to neutral.
3. Turn the head sideways and look behind you to both sides. Try to look as far behind you as possible. Do this at least 5 times and then come back to neutral.
4. Drop the right ear to the right shoulder to stretch the left side of the neck. Hold the stretch for at least 10 seconds and then repeat by bringing the left ear to the left side.
5. Return the head to neutral.

Finish by doing neck rolls.

1. Drop the chin to the chest.
2. Turn your head to the left while keeping your chin as low as it can go. The chin will get to the point where you are looking over your left shoulder.
3. Raise your chin to look up to the ceiling. *Do not drop your head back—it will compress the connective tissue between the bones in the spinal column!*
4. Think of lifting your head and neck as you turn your head to the right side, to the point where you look over your right shoulder.
5. Drop the chin and return to the middle. Continue in this direction at least 5 times then stop, and go the other way the same number of times.

Hockey

Hockey players have to worry about bodies, sticks, a hard puck, immovable walls, and the hard ice. They can get injuries from collisions with these objects. The hockey player has to pay special attention to the low back, hips, groin, shoulders, and legs. Goalies will massage and stretch the groin for the flexibility to get down and cover the ice in front of the net. The massager must take into account that hockey players usually hold the sticks on one side, so the opposite traps and shoulders are raised higher.

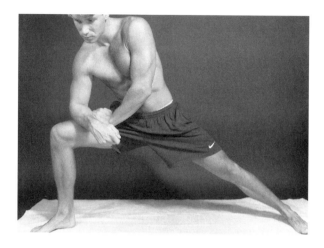

To stretch the groin and hip:

1. Stand with the legs out to the sides, shoulder-and-a-half width apart.
2. Bend the right leg and lean to the right side. The right leg is now bent. The upper body is sitting back so the knee does not go over the right toe. The left leg is out straight to the left. The stretch is for the left adductors and the right hip. Hold the stretch for at least 10 seconds, repeat, and then repeat on the other side.

Another stretch is as follows:

1. Start with the legs out to the side over a shoulder-and-a-half width. The knees are bent, the feet pointing to the front.
2. Drop the upper body down to the ground, keeping the legs in place.

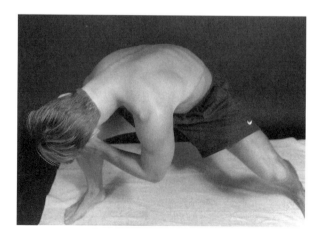

Hold the stretch for at least 10 seconds and then return the upper body to an upright position.

3. Repeat the stretch, but this time lower the upper body to the right knee. Hold, return up to an upright position, and repeat on the other side.

The lunge stretch is also included (see illustration on page 58). The athlete will do extra massage to the low back, hips, shoulders, and legs.

Martial Arts

Martial artists, like dancers, use their entire bodies. They will get injuries from the extreme range of motion of some of the movements. A martial artist's body must be very warm and flexible to avoid injuries. This does not take away from the fact that martial arts is a contact sport. These athletes will get injured from trauma. A martial artist will get the entire body. Each style has a different emphasis and must be taken into account: judo has throwing, so the low back and twisting will be a focus of the pre-event sports massage; tae kwon do emphasizes the legs, so the legs and lower back will be the focus. Work the areas that are highlighted. Another way to find these areas is to take a few classes and find where you feel the stress of the workouts the next few days after the practice. The areas that are sore are the focus areas.

A stretch for the back and shoulders is as follows:

1. Stand with the feet shoulder-width apart, the arms over the head.
2. The hands are crossed so the right hand is on the left side and the left is on the right side. The palms are facing each other. The fingers are interlaced.
3. Breathe in. Then breathe out as you lean the upper body to the right. Hold the stretch for at least 10 seconds. Come back to neutral: the starting point.
4. Breathe in. Then breathe out as you repeat the stretch to the left.

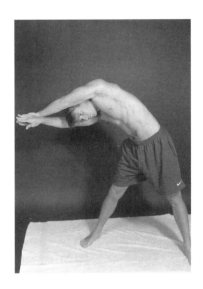

Gymnastics

Gymnasts must worry about all types of injuries to the entire body. These athletes can hold their upper body up with the shoulders out to the side as in the iron cross. They catapult in the air in tumbling techniques. In general, the ankles, foot, shin, low back, shoulder, elbow, and wrist are focus areas for injuries. Because of this, gymnasts must massage the entire body. If the athlete is only doing one or two events, the events they are doing will affect the massage. For a floor routine, balance beam, and vault, the athlete will focus the massage more on the body below the chest, even though the shoulders and arms are massaged. The uneven bar, rings, and parallel bars have the athlete focus on massaging the shoulders and arms, even though the legs and back are massaged. Gymnastics events are usually shorter then most dances, but are extremely explosive, so a gymnast should get extra massage to get the body primed for that short time period. The ankle is an important area for landing, so range-of-motion techniques are great here.

Skiing

Skiers must be careful of injuries to the hand, wrist, shoulder, low back, hips, and knees. A skier must be aware of the terrain and elements they are doing their event in. Be careful of frostbite. Downhill skiers will massage their legs and lower back. The thigh and hips are very important in staying low and getting off that outside ski. Slalom racers should also get their arms and shoulders to help take the blow from the breakaway poles. Nordic or cross-country skiers will work the shoulder and back to get the areas that help when the upper body propels them.

A stretch for the lower back is as follows:

1. Sit on the ground, the bottoms of the feet together in the middle, with the knees out to the side. The hands are around the feet or ankles.

2. Breathe out as you pull your upper body to your feet. Hold the stretch for at least 10 seconds at the lowest point.

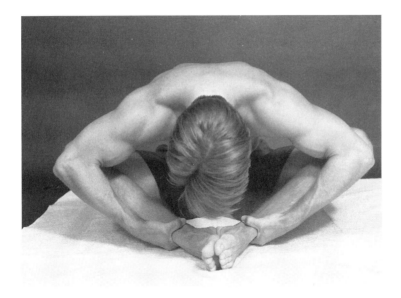

A second stretch is:

1. Sit on a chair, the right leg crossing the left leg, the right foot over the knee. The right knee is pointing to the right side.
2. Push the right knee down to the ground and feel the stretch in the butt. Hold the stretch for at least 10 seconds and repeat on the other side.

A massage stroke that a skier can do is to pat and rub the legs. She pats the legs vigorously down the outside and up the inside of the leg. After doing this cycle 5 times, she leans forward and rubs (smoothes) the lower back with both hands on their respective side.

Soccer

A soccer athlete has to worry about injuries to the legs and neck. Shin-splints, sprained ankles, hamstring pulls, and overuse foot injuries are common. In soccer, the athlete changes speeds and moves in all directions. These athletes must have good low back and leg strength and endurance. A soccer player will focus the massage on her legs and hips. A goalie, the only position where she can use her hands, will massage the shoulders and legs. A soccer player should also massage the neck and traps for all the heading of the ball that she might do.

Swimming

Swimmers need that great shoulder flexibility and endurance depending on the events or group of events they are competing in. Swimmers must worry about overuse injuries to the shoulders. Individual medley (IM) swimmers (swimmers who do all four strokes: back, breast, fly, free) need to condition and massage for all the strokes. A freestyler will work the shoulder and lats. A fly person will work the shoulders and hips. A breaststroke person will work their forearms, inner thighs, shoulders, and lats.

Stretch the chest and front shoulder (shown in basketball). To stretch the middle back:

1. Start in a sitting or standing position.

2. Cross your arms and give yourself a hug.

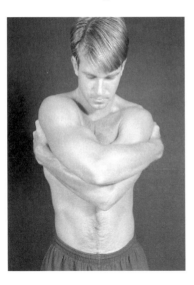

3. Squeeze the arms so that they move away and the back arches. Feel the stretch in the middle of the back between the shoulder blades. Hold the stretch for at least 10 seconds.

4. Repeat, but change arms so the second arm is over the first one.

Volleyball

Volleyball players need lightning quickness and jumping ability. Volleyball players can get injuries from being hit by the ball, as in jammed finger, or from landing improperly, as in sprained ankles. The athlete needs to have great shoulder movement to spike a ball. Emphasize the legs, arms, shoulders. Work the inner and outer hips and thighs for quick lateral motion.

Weight Lifting

A weight lifter should get the entire body, but if you are breaking the body down to body parts or areas, massage those areas. An example of this would be to lift back and biceps in one workout. You will pre-event massage the back and biceps. It is also good to do some compressions or kneading to the muscle between the sets. Shaking the muscles is a must! So after the first set of bench presses, you would compress the chest, knead the deltoids and triceps, or shake the area for a few seconds until you start your next set. Another great one is to stretch after the massage between sets, or just stretching. In the case of the bench press, stretch the chest, shoulders, and triceps, then continue with the second set. The massage will fill in the time between the sets and help you rest and rejuvenate enough to have great success in the next set. The muscles will also get the benefit of the massage. Stretch and massage the muscles that are lifting the exercise or movement.

Rowing and Kayaking

Rowing is an exercise that takes the entire body. The injuries that rowers can get are overuse injuries and muscle strains. Kayaking uses the upper body to move and the lower body usually stays stationary. Kayakers can get overuse injuries to the shoulders and stiffness in the lower back. Rowers and kayakers use the shoulders, back, chest, wrists, and upper arms a lot. These are the areas that will be emphasized. While moving along, these athletes can take a break and shake out the tight muscle areas like weight lifters. Twisting movements for the torso are great to loosen and warm this vital area. Also, one may use the cramp techniques in the maintenance chapter.

Remember to use common sense and get the area that you individually need. If you get sore or tired in a certain area, work that area with massage before the event even if I did not say to get that area for your sport. It is your body and only you know how it feels and what really helps. The above guidelines are just that—guidelines. Have fun, and good luck.

Post-Event Self Sports Massage

In post-event self sports massage, you will start the massage after you have completed your cooldown (aerobics and stretching). The goal of post-event sports massage is to cool down and replenish the body. Take off your shoes. If no stroke depth or pace is mentioned, assume they are medium to light. Use stretches where appropriate. Substitute range-of-motion techniques for the stretches once in a while. Make sure the strokes and techniques are comfortable. Take a look at pages 91–103 for sports-specific postevent massage tips.

Back, Butt, and Hips

1. Lie on your back with your hands at your sides, legs straight up in the air. To make this easier, you can bend your knees or place your legs up on a wall.

2. Stay in this position for at least 1 minute. Take deep breaths into the abdomen (instead of chest breathing). Breathe in as the abdomen extends out. Breathe out as the abdomen contracts in. Make the breaths longer and deeper into the abdomen: inhale, hold, exhale, hold. The deep breathing will release tension, replace carbon dioxide with oxygen, and give you something to focus on. Holding your legs up in the air will let gravity help bring the blood back to the heart.

3. After 1 minute, move away from the wall, place both your arms around your bent knees (bend at the knees if they are straight), and pull the knees to your chest as you keep your head on the floor. Feel the stretch in your lower back. Hold the stretch for at least 10 seconds.

4. Rock your body back and forth slightly. Rock back by pulling your legs into your chest to expose your butt. Pull up on your upper body as you release the legs slightly to expose the upper back.

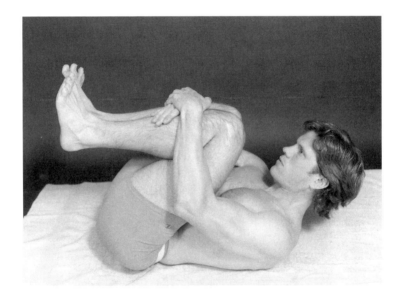

5. Finish by stopping the rocking motion and then straightening the legs onto the floor.

6. Roll onto your right side. Your right arm is bent with the right hand underneath your head. The right leg is straight out below you. The left

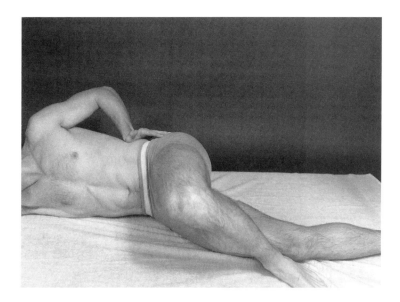

leg is bent with the knee on the ground in front of you and the left foot behind the right knee.

7. Take your left hand and place on the left low back area.

8. Smooth the lower back down from the ribs to the butt for 10–20 seconds with the palm of your hand.

9. Place the heel of the left hand onto the lower back by the ribs and do some circular compressions around the area from ribs to butt to spine. Start with light pressure and go to medium pressure for about 10 seconds.

10. Place the right hand on your left knee. Try to keep the knee on the floor with the left hand as you stretch the lower back by twisting the upper body to the left. Hold for at least 10 seconds and then repeat the stretch of the lower back (see Chapter 6).

11. Move back to your right side and knead the left butt between the heel and fingers of your left hand. Work all around the left butt from the outside hip (greater trochanter of the femur area) to the back bone (sacrum) up to the lower back.

12. After you go around the butt a few times and the muscles warm and loosen, go around once more with slow, held, kneading strokes.

13. Finish by smoothing the area with the palm of your hand.

14. Roll onto your back with your left knee in the air, the left leg bent at the knee, and the left foot on the ground.

15. Place the right foot across the left knee so the right knee falls out to the right side. The inner thigh is now facing you. This is like the piriformis stretch in Chapter 6.

16. Interlace the fingers behind the left hamstrings and pull the left leg up to your chest. You will feel the stretch in the right butt cheek. To increase the stretch, press down with your right forearm onto the right inner thigh. As you pull the legs to your chest, hold the stretch for at least 10 seconds and then slowly release.

17. Pull the leg further, hold, and then release. Try to stay on your back, relax the neck, and breathe.

18. Straighten the left leg and place it on the ground.

19. Bend the right leg so the knee is in the air, the right foot flat on the ground.

20. Place both hands on the right hamstrings.

21. Knead the right hamstring from knee down to hip. Knead the hamstring by the hip more than the lower hamstring. The hamstring muscle bellies are more in this region than lower by the knee.

22. Finish the hamstrings by smoothing them at a medium pace with the palms of your hands. Get the entire back of the thigh from knee to hip.

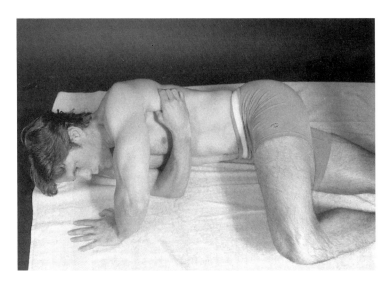

23. Roll onto your right side with the right leg straight. The left leg is bent with the left knee on the ground in front of the right leg, which is for support.
24. Knead the left side of the trunk with your right hand up from your hip to your armpit.
25. Slowly raise and lower your left arm slightly as you knead to stretch the muscles there. Stop after at least 3 times while massaging at a medium pace and pressure.
26. Finish by smoothing the area with long, slow strokes by your right hand.

Shoulder and Upper Arm

1. Lie on your left side or on your back.
2. Reach over and grab the right shoulder with your left hand.
3. Knead the right shoulder and upper arm (biceps and triceps muscles). Start the kneading on the back of the shoulder, down the triceps to the elbow, around to the outside of the upper arm, up the outside upper arm to the outside shoulder, to the front of the shoulder, and down to the front of the upper arm. Go at a slow pace and get the tissue nice and loose (see illustration on page 51).
4. After doing this cycle back and forth at least 3 times, finish by shaking around the upper arm area as if you were waking someone. Feel the tissue move as you shake the muscles of this area.

Forearm

1. Begin either sitting up or lying down.
2. Smooth up and down the right forearm with long, slow strokes. Use the palm side of your left hand. Move the smoothing around the forearm to get the entire forearm: back, sides, and front.
3. Knead the entire forearm and hand with the left hand at a medium pace. Do this in long lines from elbow to the start of the fingers.
4. After going over the forearm 2–3 times this way, grab and hold the muscles in your hand. Grab the inside and outside of the forearm and hands.
5. Shake the top of the back and front right forearm with the left hand pressed into the muscles.

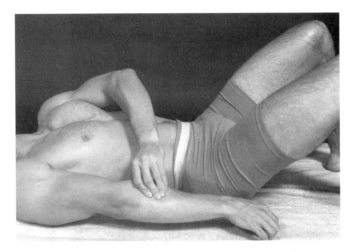

6. Finish the arm by smoothing lightly up and down the entire arm from hand to shoulder.

Roll over and do the other side.

Lower Back

1. Lie on your right side.
2. The left arm is around the chest at nipple level in front of your body.
3. The right arm is bent at the elbow with thc right hand underneath the head.
<u>**4.**</u> The arms press the upper body up as the legs stay together and on

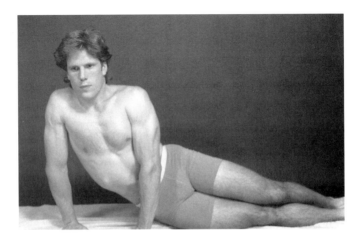

the ground so the body becomes a V. Breathe out as you bend up. This stretches the right lower back. Hold the stretch for at least 10 seconds.

5. Roll over and repeat on the other side
6. Roll on your back.
7. Take a deep breath in and breathe out as you sit up. The legs are straight in front of you.
8. Place the arms behind you with the elbows straight.
9. Lean the upper body back as you move the arms further away from the body. The stretch is felt in the front shoulders and chest.

Neck

1. Lie on your back with your knees in the air, your feet on the ground.
2. Place the fingers of both hands on the back of your neck: the right on right side and the left on left side.
3. With slow circles, circular friction the back of the neck muscles. Massage the area from the back of the head to the base of the neck. Repeat at a medium pace and depth at least 3 times.
4. Bring the right ear to the right shoulder as you pull the head to the right gently with the right hand. This will stretch the left side of the neck. Hold the stretch for at least 10 seconds.
5. Return the head to neutral.
6. Bring the left ear to the left shoulder and pull gently with the left hand to stretch the right side of the neck. Hold the stretch for at least 10 seconds.
7. Return the head to neutral.
8. Repeat on the left side, but now angle your chin up to the front of the right shoulder. This stretch will need to lift the head slightly off the ground. The back right part of the neck feels the stretch.
9. Bring the head back to center on the ground.
10. Stretch the right side by bringing the chin to the front of the left shoulder.

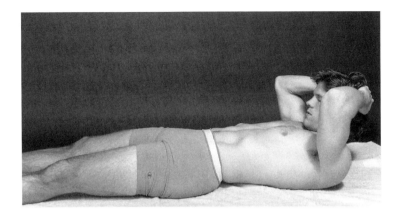

11. Stretch the back of the neck by placing the hands on the back of the head and bringing your chin to the chest. Hold all the stretches for at least 10 seconds.

12. Release the neck stretch and bring the head back to the floor.

Traps

1. Lie with your back on the ground.

2. Grab the left traps with the right hand on the side of the base of the neck (see illustration on page 50).

3. Knead the trap muscle from the neck to the edge of the shoulder with the fingers. The thumb is to the front of the traps muscles and the four fingers are to the back. The pace and depth of the massage is medium.

4. Finish by smoothing the entire area slowly.

5. Repeat on the right side with the left arm.

Chest

1. Lie with your back on the ground.

2. Make a fist with the right hand.

3. Place the heart of the fist (the palm of the fist with the fingers bent in) on the left chest muscle (see illustration on page 49).

4. Press the right heart of the fist into the chest muscle with the help of the left hand.

5. Compress, starting at the top of the left side of the sternum and move out to the shoulder. From the shoulder, compress down to the nipple on men and to the top of the breast on women. From the nipple area, compress into the sternum.

6. Complete the circle by compressing up to the starting point just off the left side of the sternum. Compress the chest muscles in a circle at least 3 times at a medium pace and medium pressure.

7. Now open the right fist and press the palm of the right hand on the chest muscle.

8. Press into the tissue with the heel of the palm and make circular strokes while not moving over the skin. Do the entire area at a medium pace and depth least 3 times. Follow the path of the chest compressions at a medium to light pressure and a medium speed.

9. Finish the chest muscles by smoothing the entire area with the right hand. The strokes are with the palm side of the hand, at a slow pace and light pressure. The strokes can go across the body from sternum to shoulder and back again.

Quads

1. Moving to the legs, take a deep breath in and breathe out as you sit up.

2. Bend the right leg so the foot is by the left knee. The left leg is straight.

3. Place the palm side of both hands on the left quads up by the hip. The right hand is on the inside of the thigh and the left is on the outside of the thigh.

4. Smooth the entire upper thigh in long, slow strokes from the hip to knee and back again. The pressure is very light.

5. Press the heels of the hands down by the knee. The left hand is on top of the thigh and the right is just on the inside of the left hand.

6. Compress the quad muscles with the heel of the hand up to the hip and back down to the knee at a medium pace and medium pressure at least 3 times. Move the hands outward so the left is on the outside of the thigh and the right is toward the top of the thigh. Repeat the compression strokes at a medium pace and medium pressure at least 3 times (see illustration on page 27).

7. Compress the heel of the right palm into the thigh on the inside of the thigh and the left hand on the outside of the thigh by the knee.

8. Circular friction the entire quad area with your fingers spread from the knee to the hip with medium pace and pressure.
9. End by smoothing the leg with light, long, slow strokes.

Lower Leg
1. Position yourself in the same sitting position as in the quads section: one leg straight and the other bent.
2. Bend the left leg so that the knee is in the air and the foot is flat on the floor.
3. Interlace the fingers of both hands and clamp the hands onto the lower leg just above the ankle.
4. Slowly and lightly, smooth the lower leg up to the knee by leaning the upper body back. Slide the hands back down to the ankle and repeat at least 3 times, adding pressure. The pressure will get as deep as medium pressure.
5. Place the interlaced hands on the inside and outside of the lower leg. The right is on the front part of the bone and the left is on the muscle on the outside of the lower leg just below the knee.
6. The hands will knead (squish and press in) the muscles on the outside of the leg in and forward. Release the tension and repeat at a medium pace. Note: If you have shinsplints, only massage the lower leg toward

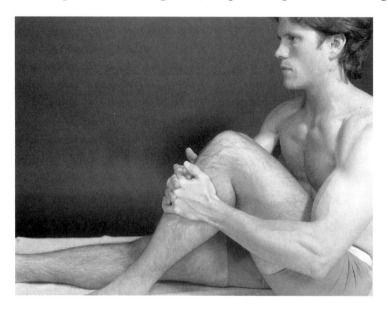

the front so that you do not pull the muscles off the tibia (a bone in the lower leg) and cause shinsplints. Repeat the stroke down to the ankle.

7. Finish the lower leg by smoothing the lower front leg up with the interlaced fingers at a medium pace and a light pressure.

8. With the fingers interlaced, pull the left knee up so the left foot is off the ground. Point the toe up to the knee and then point the toe away from your body. Repeat 3–4 times.

9. Make circles with the ankle in both directions. Do one direction 3–4 times and repeat in the other direction 3–4 times. It does not matter which direction goes first.

10. Grab the bottom of your foot (the shoes are off) with both hands. The tips of the fingers meet at the center of the sole of your foot, the left on the outside and the right on the inside of the left foot. Toes are pointed into the air. Pull the fingers apart to the side. This will spread the muscle and tissue. (Make sure not to scratch the bottom of the foot with your fingernails.) Repeat the stroke up to the toes and down to the heel at least 3 times.

11. Pull back all the toes toward your body to stretch the muscles in the bottom of your foot.

12. Straighten the left leg.

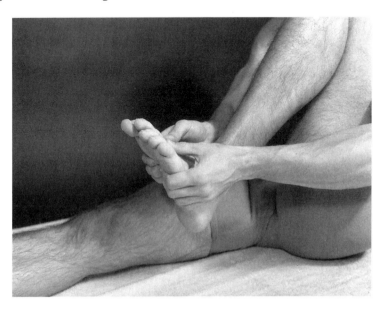

13. Drop the left knee out to the floor so the left foot faces the right knee.
14. With the right fist, knuckle the sole of the left foot from heel to toes. Repeat the stroke at least 5 times to warm the fascia and stretch it.
15. Repeat the quads and lower leg and foot on the other side.

Hamstrings
1. Lie on your back with the right leg straight on the ground, the left bent with the knee up by the chest.
2. Place the palms of both your hands by the left knee on the left leg.
3. Smooth up the leg to the left butt.
4. As you smooth the muscle, drop the knee toward the ground. The knee might only go to a right angle (90 degrees) to the floor as the hands get to the butt. Repeat the medium pressure and pace at least 3 times.
5. Bring the knee back to your chest and interlace the fingers.
6. Squeeze the hamstrings with the heels of your hands from the sides, inside with the right and outside with the left, just below the butt. Squeeze into the tissue and lift the tissue away from the bone ever so slightly. Release and let the muscle relax for a few seconds. Then repeat the procedure as you move up the leg to the knee. After 3 quarters of the way to the knee, you will have passed the bellies of the muscles on

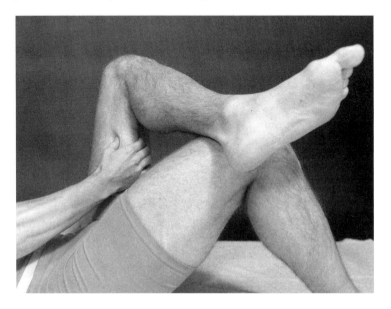

the outside of the leg. At this point, put more emphasis on the inside of the hamstrings. Finish this stroke at the knee.

7. Bend the right knee up with the right foot on the floor.
8. Cross the left ankle over the right knee and drop the left knee out to the outside
9. With your right hand, knead down and up the hamstrings from the knee. Repeat the stroke at a medium pace and medium depth.

Calves

1. The right leg is bent at the knee and the foot is flat on the ground. The left leg is bent at the knee and the left ankle is crossed over the right knee.
2. With both hands between the legs, grab the calves up by the knee and knead the back of the lower leg from knee to heel. As you go down the lower back leg, it is easier to grab with the same hand (in this case the left) than with the opposite one (see top illustration on page 41).
3. With the right fist, compress the calves from knee to heel. Avoid the areas right behind the knee cap and in line with the knee joint. This area behind the knee is where the nervous and circulatory systems run and are exposed. Start off with light compression strokes and gradually deepen them to medium as the tissue warms.
4. End by lying on your back.
5. The right leg stays bent with the foot flat on the floor, the left leg is bent but held up.
6. With both hands, smooth the lower calf area from the heel to the knee.

STRETCHES

Infraspinatus

1. Stand and place the left arm straight across the body at nipple or armpit height.
2. With the right arm, hook the left arm above the elbow with the right front elbow region. The left arm is now locked into the right arm (see illustration on page 55).
3. Using the right arm, pull the left arm toward the right side. Feel the stretch behind the shoulder on the outside of the left shoulder blade.

Hold the stretch for at least 10 seconds, repeat if necessary, and then repeat on the other side.

Triceps

1. Reach and place the left hand on the top of the left shoulder.
2. Place the right hand on the left elbow.
3. Push the left arm back and up to the ceiling while keeping the left hand in contact with the shoulder. Do not arch the back. This is done by tightening the abdominals. Hold the stretch at the highest point or at the deepest stretch for at least 10 seconds (see top illustration on page 56).
4. Repeat the stretch if necessary and then repeat on the other side.

Traps and Infraspinatus

1. Place the back of the left hand on the same side of the lower back. The left elbow is out to the side.
2. Reach across the body with the right arm and grab the left elbow.
3. Pull the elbow to the opposite (right) side. Make sure that the shoulders do not rise (see middle illustration on page 56).
4. To increase the stretch, drop the head to the side that the arm is being pulled to: for a left side stretch, the right arm is pulling the left arm to the right side and the head drops to the right. Hold the stretch for at least 10 seconds.
5. Repeat the stretch if necessary and then repeat the sequence on the other side.

Lats

1. Keep standing with the feet past shoulder-width apart for support.
2. Lean to right as you raise the left arm over your head and to the right. Feel the stretch on the outside of the back. Hold for at least 10 seconds (see bottom illustration on page 56).
3. Repeat the stretch if necessary. Then do the other side.

Low Back

1. Lie on your back with your arms out to the sides.

2. The legs are bent at the knees. The knees are straight up in the air.
3. Drop the knees to the right side so the body twists. The knees are by or on the ground. Try to keep your back flat on the ground. Hold the stretch for at least 10 seconds (see illustrations on page 65).
4. Repeat the stretch then repeat again on the other side.

Hips

1. Sit on the ground cross-legged.
2. Lift the right leg and place the right foot on the outside of the left knee. The right knee is now pointing in the air.
3. With the left arm grab the right knee and pull the upper body toward the right knee. Feel the stretch in the hips and the top of the butt on both sides.

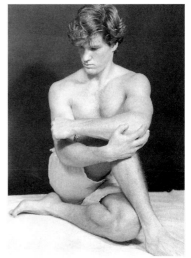

SPORTS-SPECIFIC POST-EVENT SELF MASSAGE TIPS
Running, Hiking, Jogging

In any type of running, hiking, or jogging event—the hurdles, sprints, marathons, or jogging—the massager will spend most of the time on the legs, butt, abs, and lower back. The massager will stretch the same areas: legs, butt, and trunk (all around the midsection). If the event is high intensity running or hiking, as in sprinting, hurdles, or heavy backpacking, the massager will massage and stretch the shoulder, chest, and upper back. The athlete starts by taking off his shoes. The athlete takes 3–4 deep breaths to relax himself. The athlete shakes out the ankles to loosen the lower leg muscles. The athlete can do circular compressions, smoothing, or shaking and jostling to the abs, low back, butt, quads, hamstrings, calves, and front lower leg. The pace of the strokes are slower and more rhythmic than in pre-event sports massage.

The athlete may have run for a long time and/or a great distance. Make sure the athlete rehydrates himself and takes the time to loosen the body.

These athletes should do lunge stretches, groin stretches, calf and soleus stretches, ankle and hip range of motions, and smoothing and shaking the body from below the ribs. The lunge stretch, groin stretch, calf stretch, and soleus stretch are shown in the pre-event chapter. A range of motion for the hip starts:

1. Lie down with the legs raised and the knee bent to 90 degrees.
2. The leg is circled up to the outside, to the chest, down the inside, and around in circles at least 5 times.

One other great stretch for a runner in a postevent sports massage is the standing tibialis anterior stretch.

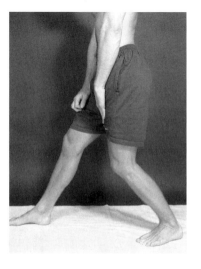

1. The athlete stands with the feet shoulder-width apart. If the runner has trouble with his balance, stand by a wall, tree, or other person to hold you up.

2. Cross the right foot over the left foot in front of you so your right toes are touching the ground.

3. Bend your left knee so the left leg pushes the right leg forward. The stretch is then felt in the front of the right leg between the knee and the ankle. Hold the stretch for at least 10 seconds and repeat on the other side. The massage strokes are long and slow.

Tennis and Racquetball

The massager will spend most of his time on the shoulder, forearms, groin, hamstrings, and calves. He will also stretch these areas. The massager can do circular compressions, smoothing, and shaking and jostling to the legs, trunk, and shoulders before a match or practice. The strokes are long and slow. The athlete does wrist and ankle rotations or shakes to cool down these vital areas.

Great stretches for these athletes are the lunge and groin stretch shown in pre-event running. For massage, the athlete can also knead the shoulders and upper arms with his hands. The strokes are slower and more rhythmic than the pre-event sports massage strokes. Use the kneading, circular palm strokes, and slow compressions to work the muscles and pump out the waste products. Circular compression strokes are great to do on the front and outside thigh while sitting in a chair. Other great areas to massage are the lower back, trunk (twisting stretches), shoulder range of motions, and wrist shaking.

Baseball

The athletes should get the neck, traps, shoulder, upper arm, elbow, forearm, wrist, and hand. The lower back and hamstrings should also be emphasized. Do the stretches in the pre-event chapter for the arms, shoulder, chest, and back. A pitcher will massage the arms and shoulder with kneading, compression, and smoothing strokes. A catcher will massage and stretch out his quads, hamstrings, and lower back. The first baseman will stretch and massage the arms and legs with particular attention to the hamstrings and groin to increase his catching reach. The side that a baseball player uses

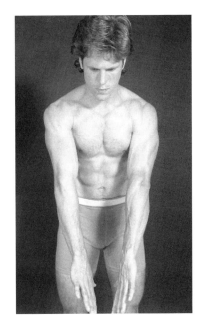

will get the most attention in stretching and massage, but, as for any training, the other side must get worked on. Another great stretch for baseball players is the press-up, so the press-up stretch should also be done. These athletes can also do shoulder and neck movements. For the shoulders:

1. Stand up with the feet shoulder width apart.
2. Round the back and bring the shoulders in. Think of trying to have them touch in the center of your chest. Hold the stretch or just do this as a movement.
3. Arch your back so the shoulders now go to the back. Think of having the shoulder blades touch in the center of the back. Hold the stretch or just do these as movements.
4. Shrug the shoulders up and down.
5. Move the shoulders in the largest circles forward and backward. Do all stretches and movements with your breath.
6. If the shoulder or elbow is sore, then do ice massage (shown in Chapter 8) to the area.

Basketball

The athlete will work the lower back, quads, hamstrings, calves, groin, feet, shoulder, and forearms. Basketball players need to spend more time in a stretch and massaging the area that is stretched because of the large number of games that they play. In one lower back stretch:

1. Lie on the ground.
2. Bring the right knee to the chest. The right knee is bent. The stretch is in the hamstrings and the lower back (see illustration on page 43).
3. Hold the stretch and knead the hamstrings with both hands. This kneading is repeated for each stretch of the lower body and any stretch to one side of the upper body.

Two other great stretches for basketball are for the shoulders.

1. Kneel facing a wall.
2. Place both hands on the wall in front of you, and lower your upper body. This stretches the lats, chest, and lower part of the shoulder capsule (see illustration on page 62).

The second stretch is as follows:

1. Sit on the ground with your legs out straight.
2. Place your arms behind your body and move your body forward to stretch the chest and shoulder (see illustration on page 63).

Another stretch for the tibialis anterior muscle:

1. Start with the athlete kneeling on the ground.
2. The feet are underneath the butt and pointing behind you (see top illustration on page 48).
3. Place your arms behind your body with the hands on the ground. Lean back slightly till you feel a stretch in the front lower legs. To get one side more than another, lean to the opposite side.

Bicycling

The areas that bikers will massage and stretch are the thighs (quads and hamstrings), hips, lower leg (front and back), low back, shoulder, arms, wrists, and neck. One stretch is great for the soleus muscle, hips, and low back.

1. Stand with the feet a little wider than shoulder-width apart, the arms at your sides.
2. Squat down so the butt is below the knees, upper body is by the knees.
3. Put your hands behind your head and pull your chin to your chest (see illustration on page 64). Hold the stretch for at least 10 seconds and then repeat.

Another stretch for a biker is the lunge stretch. This stretch is described in the running section (see illustration on page 58). The exercise "bookcases" is a range-of-motion technique that is great for the lower back.

1. Lie down on the ground, knees bent and in the air, feet are on the ground.
2. Drop the right knee to the right side and hold for a few seconds.
3. Drop the left knee to the right and twist to the right (see illustration on page 65).
4. Hold this position for a few seconds, raise the left leg to the beginning position, then raise the right to the beginning position.
5. Drop the left knee to the left side, hold, and drop the right knee to the left side. The knees are brought back up one at a time to the starting position. Repeat at least 5 times. Synchronize the breaths so you breathe out as the knee is dropped, and breathe in on the holding, between positions.

One important massage stroke for bikers is to jostle, tapot, knead, compress, shake, or smooth the quads and hamstrings slowly and thoroughly after the race. Be careful of hand cramps. Cramp techniques are shown in Chapter 8.

1. One great technique to massage the hand is to sit on a chair and have the hand to be worked on on your legs with the palm up.
2. Press the opposite elbow into the muscles of the hand and do circular massage strokes into these muscles.

Bowling

Bowlers must stretch out and massage certain areas after a game to loosen up overused muscles from the repetitive motions and next day soreness.

A stretch for the abdominals is as follows:

1. Sit on a chair, arms at your sides as shown in the pre-event bowling section.
2. Lean your upper body back and look up.
3. Take in a deep breath, push out your stomach, hold the breath, and breathe out slowly as you leans forward to the starting position. Breathe out slowly (at least 10 seconds) through your mouth.

To stretch out the lower back:

1. Sit on the ground with the legs straight out and spread as far away as possible to the sides.
2. Turn the upper body to the left so the left side of your body is over the left leg.
3. Lower the upper body down and away from the right side to the left leg. The left forearm is in front of the left leg and the right arm is stretched out over head to the left side. Hold the stretch for at least 10 seconds, take a deep breath in, and return to the starting position.
4. Repeat on the other side and then get both sides again. The hamstrings and hips should be stretched.

A motion and stretch routine for the shoulders and trunk:

1. Stand, the feet shoulder-width apart.
2. The arms are at shoulder height.
3. Cross the hands so the palms are facing each other, the fingers interlaced.
4. Twist the body to the left and hold at the furthest point (see illustration on page 71).
5. Twist to the right and hold at the furthest point.
6. Repeat 5 times in each direction.

A massage stroke to do for the torso is as follows:

1. Start in the standing position: feet shoulder-width apart and arms at your sides.
2. Turn your upper body to the right, reach over with a cupped left hand as far back as possible to the midsection, and press the fingers in to the abdominals.

3. Turn to the left and smooth the right side of the abdominals with your hand. Repeat the turning and stroke on the same side at least 3 times and then get the other side. Massage the inside forearm with the heel or elbow of the other hand to work out those tight wrist flexors (see illustration on page 66).

The bowler can also jostle, knead, compress, tapot, smooth, or shake the arm being used to bowl the bowling ball, the low back and legs.

Dance and Aerobics
In a dance performance, the whole body can be worked on, and the emphasis of the post-event sports massage will depend on the particular dance that was done. The entire body from the neck down: neck, shoulders, back, low back, hips, abdominals, quads, hamstrings, groin, calves, shins, and feet. For the massage, it is good to do long, slow circular compressions to the muscle areas. For stretches, dancers should hold the stretches for a long time: 1–5 minutes. A dancer usually has an established routine of stretches. In addition to your stretches, add circular compressions, jostling, shaking, and smoothing to the muscle that is being stretched before and after the stretch.

Golf
A golfer will massage and stretch the lower back, trunk, hips, shoulders, and inside of the forearm to get the wrist muscles. After a day of golf and standing, the feet are tired and sore.
1. Take off your shoes.
2. Press the heel of one foot into the bottom of the other foot. Massage the bottom of the foot with the heel with circular strokes up and down the bottom of the foot from heel to toes (see illustration on page 42).

A great stretch for golfers are the lunge stretch (shown in running—see illustration on page 58), the "bookcase" (in bowling—see illustration on page 65), and the following one for the lower back:
1. The athlete lies on his back. The legs are out straight and the arms are at his side.

2. He bends the right leg at the hip and knee so the knee is pointing straight up.
3. The right knee is now lowered to the left side so the right leg goes on top of the left leg. The back will now rise off the ground, but try to keep it flat. Hold the stretch for at least 10 seconds and then return to the starting position and repeat on the other side (see illustration on page 67).

Another way to do this stretch is:
1. Lie flat. Bend the right leg only at the hip (not at the knee), and keep the right leg straight as you lower it over the left leg to the ground.
2. The leg may not make it to the ground or you will have to lower the leg so the foot stays closer to the left foot. This stretch also gets the lower back and the iliotibial band on the outside of the leg.

The iliotibial band can also be stretched while standing up:
1. Stand straight with the feet shoulder-width apart and the arms at your side.
2. Step the right leg in front of the left leg about 3 inches away.
3. Lean the hip to the left as the left leg is planted to the ground. Hold the stretch for at least 10 seconds and repeat on the other side (see illustration on page 60).

One other great stretch is for the outside of the shoulder:
1. Stand straight up with the feet shoulder-width apart.
2. Reach your right arm over to the left shoulder.
3. The right arm is straight and horizontal to the ground.
4. The left arm hooks the right arm above the right elbow with the front of the left elbow. Pull the right arm in to the body and away from the right side. Hold the stretch for at least 10 seconds and repeat on the other side (see illustration on page 55).

A golfer will massage the areas that he must be careful not to injure: forearm, wrist, shoulder, and low back. Smoothing, swinging the arms in circles, and twisting of the body is great to do before each stroke.

Football

After the game, the athletes must heal, practice, and prepare for the next opponents. Football players can have just about any injury. They can break bones, tear muscles, have sprains, strains, bruises, scrapes, cuts, concussions, and more. The massager must deal with the soft-tissue injuries. the areas that need attention are the neck, shoulders, back, low back, quads, hamstrings, and ankle.

The massager will pay attention to the athlete's particular position when doing the post-event sports massage. The position of the player and the role of the player will affect the massage. A quarterback will massage shoulders, arms, trunk, and low back more. A running back will massage and stretch his legs, low back, shoulders, and forearms. Linemen will massage and stretch the legs, back, low back, trunk, and shoulders. Receivers and defensive backs massage and stretch their legs, back, low back, and shoulders.

Neck rolls and movements:

1. Stand or sit in a chair.
2. Start by nodding "yes." Drop the chin to the chest and then look up.
3. Do this movement at least 5 times and then come back to neutral.
4. Turn the head and look behind you to both sides. Try to look as far behind you as possible. Do this at least 5 times and then come back to neutral.
5. Drop the right ear to the right shoulder to stretch the left side of the neck. Hold the stretch for at least 10 seconds and then repeat by bringing the left ear to the left side.
6. Return to neutral.
7. Finish by doing neck rolls. Drop the chin to the chest.
8. Turn your head to the left while keeping your chin as low as it can go. The chin will get to the point where you are looking over your left shoulder.
9. Raise your chin to look up to the ceiling. *Do not drop your head back—it will compress the connective tissue between the bones in the spinal column*!
10. Think of lifting your head and neck as you turn your head to the right side, to the point where you look over your right shoulder.
11. Drop the chin and return to the middle. Continue in this direction at least 5 times then stop, and go the other way the same number of times.

Hockey

The hockey player has to pay special attention to the low back, hips, groin, shoulders, and legs. Goalies will massage and stretch the groin for the flexibility to get down and cover the ice in front of the net. The massager must take into account that hockey players usually hold the sticks on one side, so the opposite traps and shoulders are raised higher.

1. To stretch the groin and hip, lie on the ground with the legs up on a wall. The low back is pressed as close to the wall as possible.
2. The legs are dropped to the sides as far as they go. Hold the stretch for at least 1 minute to let gravity pull the legs away from each other. You can hold the stretch longer if you want.

Another stretch is as follows:
1. Stand with the legs shoulder-width apart.
2. The legs drop out to the sides as far as possible.
3. Drop the upper body down to the ground, keeping the legs in place. Hold the stretch for at least 1 minute and then return the upper body to an upright position (see illustration on page 59).

The athlete will do extra massage to the low back, hips, shoulders, and legs.

Martial Arts

A martial artist will get the entire body. Each style has a different emphasis and must be taken into account: judo has throwing, so the low back and twisting will be a focus of the post-event sports massage; tae kwon do emphasizes the legs, so the legs and lower back will be the focus. Work the areas which you can observe have been used. Another way to find these areas is to take a few classes and find where you feel the stress of the workouts the next few days after the practice. The areas that are sore or tired are the focus areas.

Gymnastics

In post-event sports massage the shoulder and traps are prime focus areas. So are the legs and lower back. In general, the ankles, foot, shin, low back, shoulder, elbow, and wrist are focus areas for injuries. Because of this, gymnasts must massage the entire body. If the athlete is only doing one or two events, the events they are doing will affect the massage. For a floor routine, balance beam, and vault, the athlete will focus the massage more on the body below the chest, even though the shoulders and arms are massaged. The uneven bar, rings, and parallel bars has the athlete focus on massaging the shoulders and arms, even though the legs and back are massaged. Gymnastics events are usually shorter then most dances, but are extremely explosive, so a gymnast should get extra massage to get the body primed for that short time period. The ankle is an important area for landing, so range-of-motion techniques are great here.

Skiing

Downhill skiers will massage their legs and lower back. The thigh and hips are very important in staying low and getting off that outside ski. Slalom racers should also get their arms and shoulders to help take the blow from the breakaway poles. Nordic or cross-country skiers will work the shoulder and back to get the areas that help when the upper body propels them.

A stretch for the lower back:

1. Sit on the ground.
2. The bottom of the feet are together in the middle, with the knees out to the side. The hands are around the feet or ankle.
3. Breathe out as you pull your upper body to your feet. Hold the stretch for at least 10 seconds at the lowest point (see illustration on page 73).

A second stretch is as follows:

1. Sit in a chair.
2. The right leg crosses the left leg with the right foot over the knee.
3. The right knee is pointing to the right side.
4. The athlete pushes the right knee down to the ground and feels the stretch in the butt. Hold the stretch for at least 10 seconds and repeat on the other side. This is the piriformis stretch on a chair instead of the ground as shown before on the pre-event massage section.

A massage stroke that a skier can do is to pat and rub the legs. She pats the legs vigorously down the outside and up the inside of the leg. After doing this cycle 5 times, she leans forward and rubs (smoothes) the lower back with both hands on their respective side. End the patting and rubbing with slow, deep smoothing in long strokes to relax the muscles.

Soccer

A soccer player will focus the massage on her legs and hips. A goalie, the only position where she can use her hands, will massage the shoulders and legs. A soccer player should also massage the neck and traps for all the heading of the ball that she might do.

Swimming

Individual medley (IM) swimmers (swimmers that do all four strokes: back, breast, fly, free) need to condition and massage for all the strokes. A freestyler will work the shoulder and lats. A fly person will work the shoulders and hips. A breaststroke person will work their forearms, inner thighs, shoulders, and lats.

To stretch the chest and front shoulder:
1. Sit on the ground, legs out in front of you.
2. Put your arms behind you and lean your whole body forward, away from the arms, until you feel the stretch. Hold the stretch for at least 10 seconds and repeat (see illustration on page 63).

Volleyball

Emphasize the legs, arms, shoulders. Work the inner and outer hips and thighs for quick lateral motion.

Weight Lifting

A weight lifter should work on the entire body, but if you are breaking the body down to body parts or areas for your workouts, massage those areas. An example of this would be after doing back and biceps in one workout. You will post-event massage the back and biceps. It is also good to do some compressions or kneading to the muscle between the sets. Shaking the muscles is a must! So after the first set of bench presses, you would compress the chest, knead the deltoids and triceps, or shake the area for a few seconds until your next set. Another great one is to stretch after the massage between sets or just stretching. In the case of the bench press, stretch the chest, shoulders, and triceps, then continue with the second set. The massage will fill in the time between the sets and help you rest and rejuvenate enough to have great success in the next set. The muscles will also get the benefit of the massage.

Rowing and Kayaking

Rowers and kayakers use the shoulders, back, chest, wrists, and upper arms a lot, so these are the areas that will be emphasized. While moving along, these athletes can take a break and shake out the tight muscle areas like weight lifters. Twisting movements for the torso are great to loosen and warm this vital area. Also, one may use the cramp techniques in Chapter 8.

Remember to use common sense and get the area that you, individually need. If you get sore or tired in a certain area, work that area with massage before the event even if I did not say to get that area for your sport. It is your body and only you know how it feels and what really helps. The above guidelines are just that—guidelines. Have fun, and good luck.

Pre-Event Partner Massage

The goals of pre-event massage are to warm, energize, and prepare the athlete to excel in the sporting event. While doing the massage, try to imagine how the massage you are giving would feel on you. It is easiest on the massager to kneel on one or both legs. Lean your body weight into the stroke to increase pressure. Be aware of the feedback that the athlete does and does not give to you verbally. Adjust your massage using the cues given to you. Do this massage after the athlete has done their own warm-up.

Pre-event partner massage starts with the athlete on his stomach. The back side of the body is worked on, then the front side. The strokes in pre-event are light to medium depth and at a quick pace. Include more stretches and shaking in the pre-event massage then the post-event sports massage.

Sports-specific pre-event partner massage tips are on pages 122–140.

Back

1. The athlete starts the massage on her stomach. Her head is to the side and the legs are out straight. The feet are out to the side or where they are comfortable. The arms are at the sides or bent at the elbow with the hands above the head. (One or both hands can be underneath the head to cushion it.)

2. The massager should move to the right side of the body.

3. Place your hands on the left side of the back, just across the spine by the left shoulder blade. *Do not press onto the spine!*

4. Compress the erector spinae muscles down with the heel of your left hand. The right hand can stay where it is or can move down with the other hand. It feels best if one hand holds the body and stays stationary while the other one does the massage. Move the hand 1–2 inches down each compression. Compress down to the top of the hip and continue back up the body. As you compress back up, move slightly to the outside of the left erector muscles. Do this 3–5 times at least. Compress at a medium pace and medium depth.

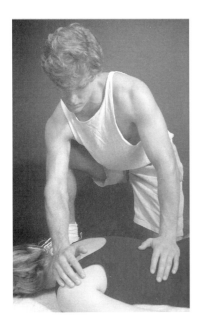

5. Finish your compressions on these muscles with light depth and a fast, invigorating pace.

6. Stop at the top by the upper shoulder blade. With the right hand compress the inside of the top edge of the shoulder blade. This is the attachment of a neck muscle (levator scapula). It may be sore, so do not work it too hard. Stay at a medium to light pace and depth. Energize the muscle. Massage the area for at least 10 seconds.

7. Compress back down the back to just above the hips. The right hand should move down to the middle of the back. Compress down into the low back muscles. Angle some of the compressions down toward the feet and up toward the head in the tissue to stretch the muscles. Work for at least

10 seconds here. Compress at a slower pace at the lower back to let the massage stroke get into all the layers of tissue. Stop every once in a while and hold the compression into the tissue to work deeper and a tiny bit longer.

Shoulder Blade

1. The athlete is on her stomach.
2. Slowly shake the athlete's body back and forth, from side to side, as you move up to the shoulder blade. Move your hands over to the left shoulder blade. It is easier to position yourself by the left hip to be angled up to the athlete's body. Compress into the left shoulder blade with the heel of your left hand. Push the shoulder blade in different directions with your compressions to loosen the musculature around the shoulder blade. Compress the outside edge of the shoulder blade below the deltoid muscle as well as on top of the shoulder blade. Compress the area for at least 30 seconds at a medium pace and a light to medium depth.

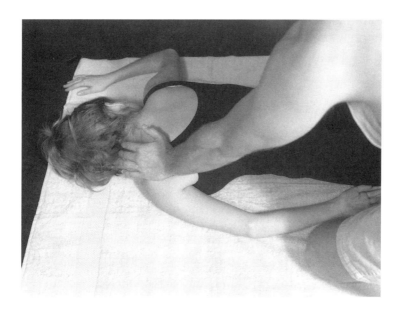

3. Grab and hold the left shoulder in your hands. The right hand is on top of the shoulder blade and the left hand is around the front of the shoulder. Using your body, move the shoulder in circles, up and down, and forward and backward. Finish by shaking the shoulder blade with the right hand to invigorate it.

Move your body to the right side and repeat the back and shoulder blade sports massages.

Neck

1. The athlete is on her stomach.
2. The massager is around either side of the shoulder area.
3. With one hand, grab the neck as one would grab the nape of the neck of a cat or dog. Slowly pull and let your fingers slide up toward you. Slowly increase the kneading (the stroke that you are doing) of the neck muscle this way from the bottom of the head to the base of the neck. Turn the head so the athlete's chin faces the other side of her body. This will help you get the muscles of the neck differently. Take about 30 seconds to massage the neck at a light depth.
4. The massager moves to the left side of the athlete's shoulder.

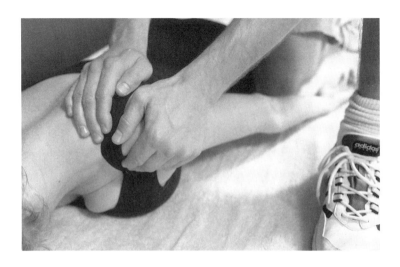

5. The massager cups the front of the deltoid muscle with his left hand and places the right hand's fingers on the inner edge of the left shoulder blade. The athlete's head is turned to the right. The massager holds the shoulder and moves his body to rotate the shoulder in circles. Circle the shoulder at least 3 times in each direction at a medium-fast pace. Do at least one large circle to stretch the muscles attached to the shoulder blade. This is like # 3 in the shoulder blade section.
6. Hold the shoulder as in #5.
7. Pull the shoulder away from the turned head and down. Hold the stretch of the neck muscles for at least 10 seconds.

Shoulder and Triceps

1. The athlete is on his stomach.
2. The massager is on the side of the body that she will work on, around ribs level. Place your hands on the shoulder and shoulder blade.
3. Compress the deltoid and the triceps. The massager will only get the back of the deltoid. Knead the deltoid for at least 10 seconds.
4. Compress down the upper back of the arm, from the shoulder to the top of the elbow. Finish the area with some brisk shaking on the muscle areas worked on here.

Repeat the neck and shoulder on the other side.

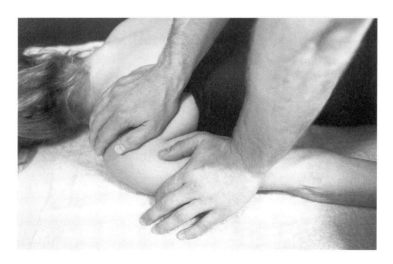

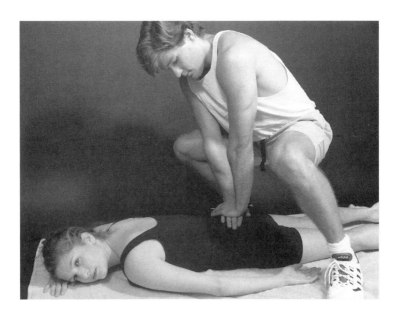

Butt

1. The athlete is on her stomach.
2. Move your body to the hips on the left side.
3. Compress into the butt with the heel of your right hand. Compress in horizontal lines and around as you get the entire butt area from the middle of the body out to the hip area. Work on the top part of the butt by the lower back. This is a major area for dancers or other athletes who stand on one leg or move from side to side. Compress for at least 30 seconds. Work at a medium pace and depth.
4. Press in with the palm and shake the muscles out with the palm of your hand at a fast pace.
5. Finish by pressing down just below the base of the spine between the left and right butt cheeks (the sacrum bone). Do this by standing over them, facing the upper body, one leg on each side, and the palms of the hands pressing the sacrum down and to the lower legs. Hold the pressure for at least 10 seconds.

Hamstrings

1. The athlete is still on his stomach.
2. The massager is on the left side, in the knee-to-hip region.

3. Place the heel of the left hand into the back thigh area. The right hand is down by the knee, either on the hamstring or just below the knee on the calf muscles.

4. Compress with the heel of your hand down the middle back thigh from the bottom of the butt to the top of the knee. Massage this area at least 3 times at a medium pace and depth.

5. Place the right heel of the hand (or a loose fist) on the inside of the left hamstring right below the butt. The left hand is down by the bottom of the hamstrings or on the top of the calf muscles.

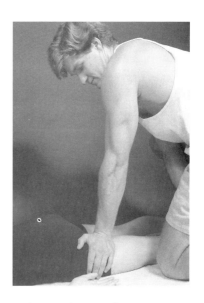

6. Compress down the inner hamstring from this starting point to the top of the inner knee. Move the hand slightly down each compression (1–2 inches). Compress at a medium pace and depth at least 3 times.

7. Turn your body toward the leg. Knead the entire hamstring area with both hands. Emphasize the upper and middle hamstrings.

8. Finish by shaking the entire area from the butt to the knee.

Iliotibial Band

1. The athlete is on her stomach.

2. The massager is on the left side by the left knee, angled toward the right shoulder.

3. The athlete brings the left knee up to the left side so the athlete's outside of the thigh is showing. *Only do this massage work if the athlete is comfortable, with no pain in the hip or knee.*

4. The massager's left hand is holding the left knee to the ground. The heel of the right hand compresses the middle of the outside of the thigh from the hip down to just above the knee. Compress down and up the thigh at a

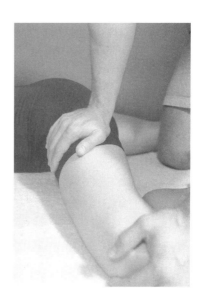

medium pace and depth (lighten the depth if the massage is painful) at least 3 times.

5. Finish by smoothing down the thigh 2–3 times at a light and fast pace and depth.

6. Bring the leg back to a straight position so the hamstrings are again showing.

Quad Stretch

1. The athlete is still on her stomach.
2. The massager is positioned on the left, between the knee and the hip.
3. With the right hand, grab the front of the left ankle.
4. Bend the lower leg so the heel of the left foot goes to the butt.
5. Move the leg in slowly till the athlete feels the stretch in the front of the left thigh. The heel of the foot may be pressed into the butt. Hold the stretch for at least 10 seconds. Sometimes it is great to hold the stretch for a few minutes so the athlete can really feel the stretch.
6. Release the stretch slowly and return the foot to the floor. The stretch may be repeated.

Hip Flexor Stretch

1. The athlete and the massager are in the same position as in the quad stretch.
2. The massager is kneeling on one leg, the right further forward than the left.
3. Bend the athlete's right knee to decrease the angle between the foot and the butt with the left hand.
4. Place her right foot on the front of the left shoulder.
5. Grab the inside right knee with the left hand. The right hand presses into the middle of the right butt.
6. Lift the right knee up off the ground by leaning forward to the right leg. The knee may go about 0–4 inches up off the ground depending on the athlete's flexibility. To keep the lower back from arching, the massager tells the athlete to contract the abdominal muscles. Hold the stretch for at least 10 seconds. Hold longer if this area is tight or the athlete has lower back problems.
7. Release the stretch slowly and bring the knee to the ground.
8. Keeping your hold on the foot, lift the leg off the ground slightly to drop

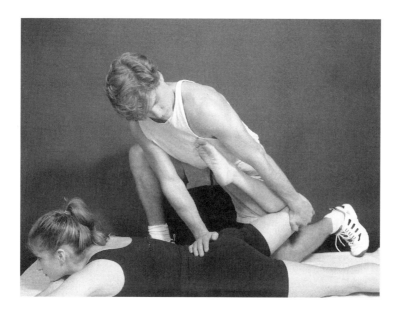

the leg to the ground. Raise and drop the leg at a fast pace so the leg hits the ground gently. This action lets the ground tapot the front of the thigh. Do this for at least 10 seconds.

9. Stop the tapotment and lower the foot to the ground.

Calves

1. The athlete is still on his back.

2. The massager is on the right, between the knee and the foot.

3. Place the right heel of your hand on the inside left calf muscle just below the knee. The left hand is immobile on the outside of the top right knee.

4. Compress with the heel of the hand or a loose fist down to above the left heel of the foot. Make sure that the athlete's foot is comfortable. Move up and down this area 3 times with constantly deeper pressure till you get to a medium depth. The pace is also medium throughout.

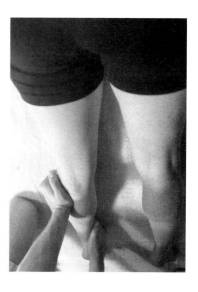

5. Repeat the compressions on the outside of the calves. Now keep the right hand down by the ankle as the left hand compresses the area from below the knee to the ankle.

6. After doing the compressions 3 times, knead the area with both hands. Especially get the top three-quarters of the lower leg.

7. Finish by shaking the entire lower leg vigorously.

Tibialis Anterior Stretch

1. The athlete is on her back with her legs straight out.

2. The massager is down by the right foot.

3. Grab the right foot with your right hand and the top of the back of the ankle with your left hand. Put the front ankle on your kneeling left knee (see illustration on page 155).

4. Pull the foot so the toes go away from the body (as in pointing; plantar flexion). Have the athlete feel the stretch on the front of the lower leg. Hold the stretch for at least 10 seconds.

5. Finish the stretch by releasing slowly. Lower the foot and leg to the ground.

Feet

1. The athlete is on his stomach with the legs out straight. IIis shoes are off.

2. The massager is below the athlete's feet, facing up the body.

3. Place your fists into the bottoms of the feet.

4. Compress the bottoms of the feet with loose fists (knuckle area). Com-

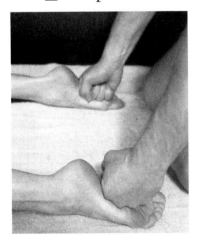

press the area from the heel to the toes. The pressure here is from medium to deep and the pace is medium. Press and hold the soft, loose fist at the bottom of the foot just in front of the ankle.

5. Finish the foot by smoothing the entire area vigorously. Do this by leaning your upper body over the feet and letting your fists slide to the toes.

Get the entire lower right extremity from the butt to the feet. Then flip the athlete over onto his back.

Chest

1. The athlete is on his back. His legs are out straight. His arms are at his sides, out from the body at a 45-degree angle. The palms are up.
2. The massager is on the athlete's left side, below the arm.
3. With your left arm grab the athlete's left arm by the wrist. Hold the arm and wrist up on your left knee, in the air, or on the ground.
4. Gently swing the arm slightly back and forth (body mobilization technique) slightly and slowly to relax the muscles. Stop after 10 seconds and then just hold the arm in the air.
5. Place the heel of your right hand on the outside of the left chest. *On women, do not press into the breast tissue.*

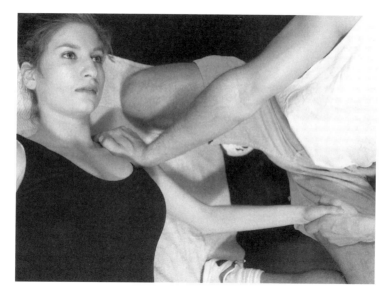

6. Compress in lines and circles from the shoulder into the middle chest (do not work on the sternum, the bone in the middle of the chest), down and back out again. Compress the entire chest area at least 3 times. The pace and depth is medium.
7. Finish the chest area by shaking the tissue with your right hand.

Front Upper Arm, Forearms, and Hands

1. The athlete is on her back and in the same position as above.
2. The massager is by the hips, facing the athlete's head.

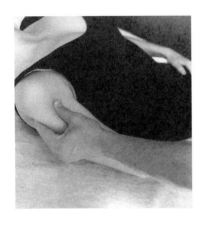

3. With your right hand, grab the athlete's right hand as if you were giving a handshake.

4. With the left hand, knead the whole deltoid muscle (shoulder muscle). Knead the area for at least 10 seconds.

5. Place the heel of the left hand on the biceps. Compress the biceps from the deltoid to the front elbow. Do this at least 3 times. Move down to the outside of the elbow.

6. The athlete's right palm is now flat on the ground.

7. Compress the outside forearm from the elbow to the wrist. Compress down and up 3 times.

8. Stop and move to the inside of the elbow.

9. The right palm is now up.

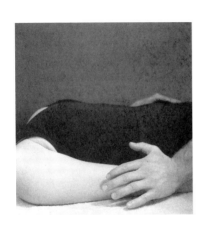

10. Compress the inside forearm from the elbow to the wrist. Compress down and up 3 times. In all of these strokes, the pace and depth is medium.

11. Move to the right hand of the athlete.

12. Her palm is up in your left hand as you massage the hand on the ground.

13. Compress around the palm of the hand with your right loose fist at least 4 times.

14. Finish the area by shaking the hands vigorously.

Neck Stretch

1. The athlete is on his back with the arms relaxed by his side and his legs straight out.
2. The massager is above the head, facing the feet.
3. Place both hands on the opposite shoulder blades so the arms are crossed. It does not matter which arm is over which. Ask the athlete to take a deep breath in and breathe all the way out slowly.
4. As the athlete breathes out, the massager lifts the head slowly so the chin of the athlete moves to touch the chest. If the athlete is too tight or the

stretch is uncomfortable, hold it at a comfortable point where he feels the stretch. Hold the stretch at its greatest point for at least 10 seconds. Remind the athlete to continue to breathe (see illustration on page 144).

5. Release the stretch by having the athlete take another deep breath in and out. Lower the head slowly as he breathes out.

6. With the head on the ground, angle yourself to the athlete's left shoulder.

7. Place your right hand on the side of the athlete's head above the left ear, and your left hand on his left shoulder.

8. Have the athlete breathe in again. Stretch the head to the right shoulder as he breathes out. Hold the stretch at its furthest comfortable point for at least 10 seconds.

9. Release the head to neutral as above, with the breath.

10. Stretch the other side.

11. Continue the process of having the athlete breathe as you stretch the neck at angles between the first one to the front and those to the sides.

12. Do the same sequence for stretching the neck to each side in rotations, left and right. To stretch the neck to the left, place your right hand on the left back of the head and the left hand on the right front side of the head.

Back Stretch

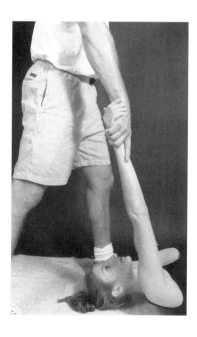

1. The athlete is on her back. The legs are out straight and the arms are relaxed by her side.

2. The massager is standing over her head, facing her feet.

3. Squat down and grab the wrist of the athlete's hands, your left in her left and your right in her right.

4. Straighten your legs as you pull on her arms to lift her upper body off the ground. The angle that her upper body makes to the ground is from 10 to 50 degrees. The athlete will feel the stretch in her back as she hangs from your arms. Hold the stretch for at least 10 seconds.

5. Lower the athlete if your hands slip on her wrists. This is overcome by having her grab and continue to hold your wrists. When she lets go, you have less to hold as her wrist tendons loosen and she slips in your hands.

6. Also do the back stretch by pulling one side of her body up higher than the other. Lower that upper side so that each is equal and then do the other side by raising it higher. You can do this by shifting your body from one side (the opposite one that you want to raise) to the other.

7. Lower her upper body to the ground slowly so the tension in her shoulders is released. Continue to hold her wrists.

8. Move her arms in small, slow circles (both directions). Repeat the circles at least 3 times to relax the shoulder musculature that helped to hold her up.

9. Finish by placing her arms at her sides on the ground.

Groin

1. The athlete is on her back. The legs are out straight and the arms are at her sides.

2. The massager is on the right side of her by the knees.

3. Bring the right leg up and out so the knee is off the ground to the outside and the sole of her foot is by the other knee.

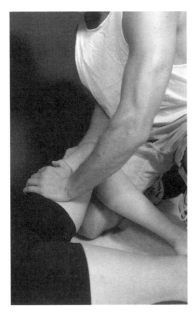

4. Place one or both of your legs by your knee underneath her knee to stabilize her leg.

5. Compress the inside of her leg with the heel of your left hand. The right hand holds the leg by the knee. The pace and depth are medium. Start with light pressure to get the gracilis muscle to loosen and then get deeper into the other adductor muscles. Compress up and down to the hip at least 3 times. Avoid the groin area and front of the hip where the leg meets the hip, which are areas of sensitive nerves and blood vessels.

6. Stop and then stretch the groin muscles by moving your legs, placing your right hand on her left hip, the left hand on her knee, and gently

pressing the knee down to the ground. Avoid pressing with the right hand into the bony points of the hip, which hurts.

7. Finish the groin by shaking the area vigorously to energize it.

Front Upper Leg

1. The athlete is on his back with the legs out straight and the arms relaxed.

2. The massager is down by his right leg, kneeling on the left leg, and with the left hand on the outside upper leg and the right hand by the knee.

3. Compress with the heel of your hand down the outside of the thigh with your left hand in straight lines from hip to knee. Do this at least 3 times.

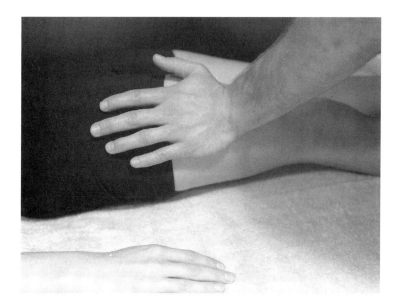

4. Move to the top of the thigh and the outside of the thigh.

5. Compress each line at least 3 times.

6. Press the outside of the right knee with your right hand to have the outside of the thigh showing to the heel of your left hand.

7. After getting the outside and top of the front thigh, hold the left hand just below the hip and compress the inside of the thigh with the heel of your left hand. Get the area from the knee to the hip. The line moves slightly to the outside or top of the thigh as the left hand compresses up the front thigh. Do this at least 3 times.

8. Stop and face the other front thigh.

9. Knead the front right thigh with both hands, from knee to hip and inside to outside, at least 3 times.

10. Finish the massage on the front thigh by shaking the thigh with both hands, the right hand on the inside and the left hand on the outside. The leg can slightly rotate from side to side, which will help release the hip muscles.

Hamstring Stretch

1. The athlete is on her back. The legs are out straight and the arms are relaxed by her side.

2. The massager is on the athlete's left side by the lower leg, facing her head.

3. Grab the left ankle above the back heel with the left hand and hold above the knee with the right to keep the entire leg straight.

4. Lift the left leg up toward the upper body to stretch the hamstring muscles. Hold the stretch at its highest point for at least 10 seconds. It is better to hold the stretch here for much longer. This muscle, if tight,

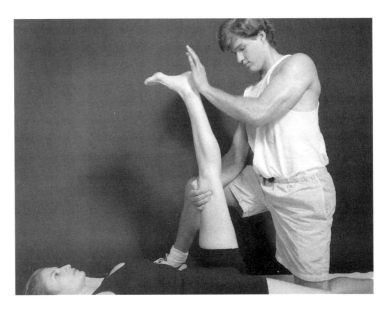

can cause a lot of lower back pain! The stretch can happen at many heights off the ground. For very tight people, the leg only has to raised a few inches off the ground. For people who are flexible, the leg has to be raised past the 90 degree mark (straight up). Be careful to keep the leg straight or the hamstring will not be stretched as much. Make sure that the other leg stays on the ground or it will loosen the stretch. Look at the same hip to make sure that the butt does not raise off the ground. To get different sides of the hamstrings, angle the leg into or away from the body about 15 degrees at the higher points of the stretch.

5. Release the stretch by bringing the leg down to the ground gently.

Front Lower Leg

1. The athlete is on his back. The legs are out straight and the arms are relaxed.

2. The massager is down by the feet, angled up toward the opposite shoulder.

3. The right hand holds the top of the ankle and the left hand is below the right knee on the muscles on the outside of the lower leg.

4. Compress the front outside lower leg with the left hand. Compress the area from the bottom of the knee to the top of the outside of the ankle.

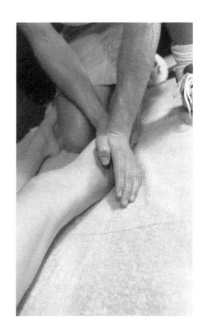

5. After at least 3 times, turn the foot in to the body with the right hand and compress in straight lines toward the outer part of the lower leg. Compress the area all the way out to the outside of the lower leg, just before the start of the calves.

6. After the compressions, grab the inside edge of the right foot with the right hand. The left hand holds the ankle and stabilizes the leg so it does not move.

7. Using the right hand, move the ankle up and

down at a medium pace so the toes of the feet point toward and then away from the body. Do this at least 3 times.

8. Stretch the ankle at the end range of motions at the top and bottom of the movements.

9. Then, using the hands in the same way, turn the foot in and out so the bottom of the foot turns in and out. (The foot turns in more than it turns out.) Do not do this or the next range-of-motion exercise on an athlete with a sprained ankle! Do this at least 3 times.

10. Then turn the ankle in the largest circles possible, with the same hand positioning. Circle both ways at least 3 times.

11. Finish the lower leg with fast light compressions on the lower leg muscles.

Repeat on the other leg.

SPORTS-SPECIFIC PRE-EVENT PARTNER MASSAGE TIPS
Running, Hiking, Jogging

In any type of running, hiking, or jogging event—the hurdles, sprints, marathons, or jogging—the massager will spend most of the time on the legs, butt, abs, and lower back. The massager will stretch the same areas: legs, butt, and trunk (all around the midsection). If the event is high-intensity running or hiking, as in sprinting, hurdles, or heavy backpacking, the massager will massage and stretch the shoulder, chest, and upper back.

The massager does ankle range of motions: circles the ankle in the largest circles, points the toes up and down, turns the ankle in and out, and squeezes the toes in and spreads them out. The massager can do circular compressions, smoothing, or shaking and jostling to the abs, low back, butt, quads, hamstrings, calves, and front lower leg.

Runners, hikers, and joggers must worry about overuse injuries, pulled muscles, and falling injuries. These injuries could include shinsplints, blisters, pulled or strained hamstrings, and sprained ankles or wrists. When falling, the athlete must worry about cuts and bruises. These athletes must be very careful of the elements—hot, cold, wet, snowy, and any other combination of weather. Also, the outside athlete must worry about dogs and other animals that could hurt them.

The massager should stretch the hips (similar to a lunge stretch), groin, calf, and soleus, and do ankle and hip range of motions. The massager should do smoothing and shaking the body from below the ribs. The strokes are fast and invigorating.

The partner lunge stretch:

1. Start out with the athlete on his back with the arms relaxed.
2. The massager bends the left leg at the knee, then lifts the leg up and pushes the knee towards the chest.
3. The end position has the athlete's knee as close to the chest as possible. The right leg does not come off the ground.
4. The massager ends the stretch by lowering the leg back to the ground.

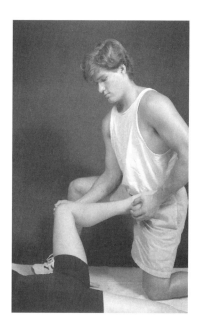

Instead of doing the stretch, the massager can just lift the leg up to the chest and lower it back down in fluid motions. This is a great hip range-of-motion technique.

The groin stretch:

1. The athlete is on her back.
2. The massager brings the right leg out to the left side as far as it will go. The massager's left leg stabilizes the right leg of the athlete's so that it does not move to the left.

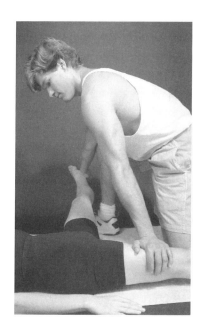

The calf stretch is best done by the athlete. Therefore, the athlete will do the same stretch as in the pre-event self massage chapter. The soleus stretch is the same, but the knee of the stretched leg is bent to get the muscle underneath. Do range of motion of the hip. Start with the athlete on her back. The knee is raised like in the hip stretch, but only till the knee points straight up. The massager then moves the leg in circles at a medium pace. The leg is moved in both directions 3–4 times.

Tennis and Racquetball

The massager will spend most of his time on the shoulder, forearms, adductors, hamstrings, and calves of the athlete. He will also stretch these areas. The massager can do circular compressions, smoothing, and shaking and jostling to the legs, trunk, and shoulders before a match or practice. The massager does wrist and ankle rotations or shakes to warm up these vital areas.

1. The massager grabs the athlete's right wrist with his left and the athlete's right wrist with his right.

2. The massager then moves the hand in circles, up and down, and across at a medium speed.

A tennis or racquetball player must be aware of overuse injuries, falling injuries, and one-sidedness injuries (most tennis or racquetball players only use one arm to hit and serve and favor the forehand or backhand). The overuse injuries happen to the shoulders, forearm extensors by the elbow (tennis elbow), and wrist. The falling injuries happen to the ankle or groin, and the one-sidedness injuries happen to the shoulder, elbow, wrist, and low back. These athletes must also be careful about being hit by the flying projectile.

Great stretches for these athletes are the hip and groin stretch shown in running. Another great stretch is the standing iliotibial stretch, shown in the pre-event massage chapter.

The partner stretch for the iliotibial band:

1. Start with the athlete on her back with the legs out straight.

2. The massager brings the athlete's right foot across the left leg by the knee.

3. The massager places his left hand on her right hip and the right hand goes to the outside of the right knee.

4. Holding the leg down with the left hand, the massager pushes the leg across the body and down to the left side. The leg will not move too far. Hold the stretch for at least 10 seconds and repeat on the other side.

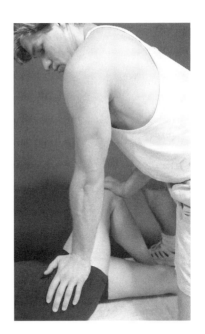

The athlete can also knead the shoulders with his hands. Other great areas to massage are the lower back, trunk (twisting stretches), shoulder range of motions, and wrist shaking.

Baseball

A baseball player uses his shoulders, upper arms, wrists, legs, and trunk when playing baseball. He needs these areas to work correctly to transfer the forces produced by the legs to work on the ball or bat. Baseball players must be careful of injuries to the elbow, forearm, wrist, shoulder, low back, and the hamstrings. All these injuries can happen from a collision with someone or the ground, or overuse by the repetitiveness of the sports (most baseball players only use one arm to throw, bat from one side, and sit behind a plate for over 3 hours).

The athletes should get the neck, traps, shoulder, upper arm, elbow, forearm, wrist, and hand massage. The lower back and hamstrings should also be emphasized. The massager should move the shoulders in all its movements. A pitcher will stretch out the arm.

The triceps stretch shown in the pre-event self massage general workout is great. Begin as for the self massage:

1. Reach and place the left hand on the top of the left shoulder.

2. Place the right hand on the left elbow.

3. Push the left arm up to the ceiling while keeping the left hand in contact with the shoulder. Do not arch the back (see top illustration on page 56).

4. The massager can grab the raised elbow to help stretch the arm more.

5. The athlete then brings both arms to the back and clasps the hands.

6. The massager will then raise the arms to the back. Hold the stretch at its highest point for at least 10 seconds, release, and repeat. This stretch stretches the front of the shoulder and the chest muscles.

The massager then does the infraspinatus stretches.

1. The athlete is standing or sitting. The athlete puts the back of his hand on his lower back (same side).

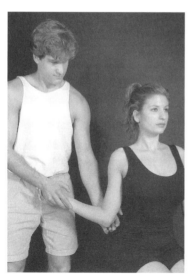

2. The massager grabs the arm at the elbow and pulls the arm forward so the athlete feels the stretch on the back of the shoulder blade.

3. The massager stretches the subscapularis muscle by having the right arm at the athlete's right side. The elbow of the right arm is bent to a 90-degree angle.

4. The massager grabs the right hand in his right hand and uses his left hand to hold the athlete's elbow at the side of the body.

5. The massager then pulls the arm away from the front of the body while keeping the elbow at his side. Hold the stretch for at least 10 seconds and then repeat.

A catcher will also stretch out his quads, hamstrings, and lower back. The first baseman will stretch the arms and legs with particular attention to the hamstrings and groin to increase the catching stretch. The side that a baseball player uses will get the most attention in stretching and massage, but, as in any training, the other side must get worked on.

Another great stretch for baseball players is the press-up. The athlete will do this by himself:

1. The athlete lies down on his stomach with his hands underneath the chest.
2. He presses up the upper body as he keeps the legs and hips on the floor (see bottom illustration on page 61).
3. Then he looks up to complete the stretch of the abdominals and front of the neck.
4. Hold the stretch for at least 10 seconds and repeat.

Basketball

A basketball player uses the entire body when she jumps, shoots, passes, twists when rebounding, and sprints when running the floor. The basketball player must get the entire body warmed and stretch out to play this game. The basketball player must contend with injuries to the ankles, shins, and lower back overuse injuries to the legs, jammed fingers, elbows to the head, and contusions from the body contact.

The massager will massage the lower back, quads, hamstrings, calves, groin, feet, shoulder, and forearms. Basketball players need to spend more time in a stretch and massaging the area that is stretched because of the large number of games that they play. The massager can do the stretches shown in the running chapter. The massager can hold the stretches and knead or compress the stretched muscles. Kneading and compressing are repeated after each stretch of the lower body and any stretch to one side of the upper body. Two other great stretches for basketball are for the shoulders.

1. First, the athlete is on her knees facing the massager.
2. The athlete bends her upper body forward (see illustration on page 62).
3. The massager grabs the athlete's hands and raises the arms above her head slowly. This stretches the lats, chest, and lower part of the shoulder capsule.

A second stretch for the shoulder:
1. The athlete stands with her legs shoulder-width apart.

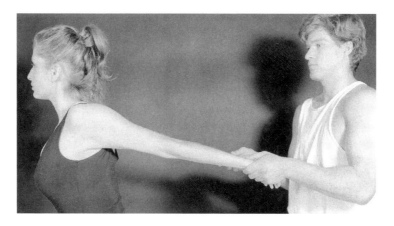

2. She then places her arms behind her body and the massager grabs the arms and pulls them up behind her to stretch the chest and shoulder.

3. The massager can grab and pull on the foot lightly to increase the stretch. Play around with the space between the arms.

A stretch for the back:

1. Start with the athlete sitting on the ground with the knees to the outside and the feet together in the middle.

2. The athlete grabs his feet and drops his head.

3. The massager, behind the athlete, pushes the upper body of the athlete slowly down to his feet. Hold the stretch for at least 10 seconds (see illustration on page 135).

Bicycling

Road and mountain bikers are athletes who go long distances and ride for a very long time. These athletes must worry about overuse injuries and falling injuries. These athletes must "sit" for long periods and thus the hamstrings and low back may be tight and cause low back pain. Bikers also get shin-splints from the toe clips, shoes, and the long period of using the ankle in only one way. Bikers also fall because of the terrain, other bikers, fatigue, or technical problems. The injuries caused by falling are to the skin of the legs, arms, and hands; shoulder and upper arm injuries from hitting the ground; and head injuries (always wear a helmet).

The areas that bikers will be massaged and stretched are the thighs (quads and hamstrings), hips, lower leg (front and back), low back, shoulder, arms, wrists, and neck. One stretch is great for the soleus muscle, hips, and low back.

1. The athlete stands with the feet a little wider than shoulder-width apart and the arms at her side.
2. She will then squat down so the butt is below the knees. Her upper body is by the knees.
3. She then puts her hands behind her head and pulls her chin to her chest (see illustration on page 64).
4. The massager can push the athlete's head forward and down to get a deeper stretch on the lower back. Hold the stretch for at least 10 seconds and then repeat.

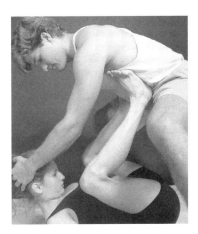

This stretch can also be done lying down, as follows:

1. The athlete is on her back with the legs out straight.
2. The massager brings the athlete's knees up to the chest and places her feet on his chest to stretch the lower back.
3. The massager then leans forward and pulls up the head to the chest with both hands. Hold the stretch for at least 10–30 seconds and then lower first the head and then the feet.

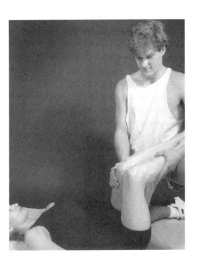

Another stretch for a biker is the partner lunge stretch, which is shown in the running section.

A modified "bookcase" range-of-motion technique is great for the lower back:

1. Starts with the athlete down on her back. The knees are bent and in the air. The feet on the ground.
2. The massager is kneeling on one leg.
3. The massager lifts the athlete's legs off the ground and places them on one leg.

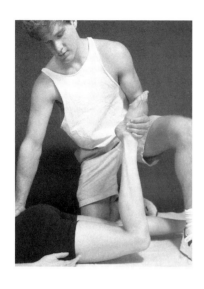

4. The massager moves the legs in circles, 3–4 in each direction, by using the body to initiate the movements.

One important massage stroke for bikers is to jostle, tapot, knead, compress, shake, or smooth the quads and hamstrings vigorously before the race.

1. To tapot the quads, the athlete lies on his stomach.

2. The massager grabs a foot and bends the athlete's knee 90 degrees.

3. The massager then raises the leg off the ground and bounces the leg on the ground at a fast pace. The floor is used to tapot the athlete's leg. Do the tapotment off the ground for at least 30 seconds.

4. Stop and then bend the ankle to the ground and hold the stretch to the soleus muscle. Lower the leg back to the ground. Repeat on the other side.

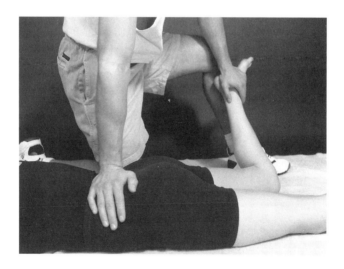

Bowling

Bowlers try to throw a heavy round object the same way 10 to 21 times a game. In bowling, the body twists, bends, and throws. The bowler usually only uses one arm to throw this heavy ball down the lane. The way the body bends and twists, along with the heaviness of the ball and the repetitiveness of the action, can help cause a trauma to the body. The low back, shoulder, hips, hamstrings, back, forearm, and wrist are all important areas.

The massager must stretch and warm the athlete's torso. Bowling is a sport, and one must prepare for bowling as such. Proper cardiovascular warm-up before pre-event sports massage is imperative. It will help the massage and stretches, help to avoid injuries, burn calories, and help your game.

A stretch for the low back:

1. Start with the athlete standing up with the feet shoulder-width apart and the arms at her sides.
2. She breathes out and leans to the right side.
3. She reaches over the body with the left arm to increase the stretch and to help stretch the lats (see bottom illustration on page 56).
4. The massager will pull the arm further away and down to get a deeper stretch. Hold the stretch for at least 10 seconds, take a deep breath in, and return to the starting position.
5. Repeat on the other side and then get both sides again.

To stretch the low back, spine, and outer thigh:

1. The athlete starts by sitting down on the ground. The legs are out straight.
2. The left foot is moved across the right leg and the foot is flat on the ground by the knee.
3. The athlete looks to the left side and behind her.
4. The massager presses his left hip into her back. He grabs the left leg of the athlete and pulls it to the right.
5. The massager also grabs the left shoulder and pulls that to the left. Hold the stretch for at least 10 seconds and repeat on the other side. The hamstrings and hips should be stretched.

Dance and Aerobics

A dancer uses her whole body. She twists, jumps, stands on her toes, holds other dancers in the air, and every other type of combination of body movements that a choreographer can think up. These athletes must really do massage, as most of them do now. They get overuse injuries and trauma from the extremeness of the movements. The whole body is worked on, and the emphasis of the pre-event sports massage will depend on the particular dance that will be done. What are the major areas that could get injured? These are the areas to massage—from the neck down—neck, shoulders, back, low back, hips, abdominals, quads, hamstrings, groin, calves, shins, and feet. For stretches, dancers should hold the stretches for a long time: 1–5 minutes. A dancer usually has an established routine of stretches. In addition to your stretches, add circular compressions, jostling, shaking, and smoothing to the muscle that is being stretched before and after the stretch.

Golf

Golf is a sport of (hopefully) long walks between a smooth, clean stroke. Unfortunately, these clean and effortless strokes don't always happen. Golf is a sport that must be done for a long period of time to master it. The games are long (9, 18, 36 holes) and in warm to hot sunny weather. Golfers get overuse and trauma injuries. A golfer must also watch out for dehydration and other weather injuries (overheating in the summer and frostbite in the winter, fall, and spring; lightning; and rain). Some major golf injuries are golf elbow (overuse or trauma to the inside forearm muscles), low back pain, and pulled muscles (hamstring, shoulder, arm, back). A golfer uses one dominant side more than the other, so one side may be overdeveloped. The stroke entails the whole body to work in unison so the ball will travel in its desired trajectory. A golfer will massage and stretch the lower back, trunk, hips, shoulders, and inside of the forearm to get the wrist muscles.

Great stretches for golfers are the partner lunge stretch (shown in the running section—see top illustration on page 123), the modified "bookcase" (in bicycling—see bottom illustration on page 129), and the following one for the lower back:

1. The athlete lies on his back. The legs are out straight and the arms are at his side.
2. The massager bends the right leg at the hip and knee so the knee is pointing straight up from the hip to the sky (see top illustration on page 123).
3. The massager presses the right knee down over to the left side so the right leg goes to the ground on the left side.

4. The massager holds the right shoulder of the athlete to the ground with her left hand. Try to keep the back flat on the ground. Hold the stretch for at least 10 seconds and then return to the starting position and repeat on the other side.

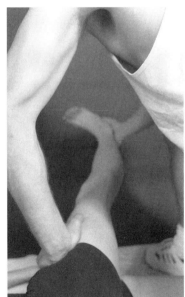

Another way to do this stretch is:

1. Lie flat. Bend the right leg only at the hip (not at the knee), and keep the right leg straight as you lower it over the left leg to the ground.
2. The leg may not make it to the ground or you will have to lower the leg so the foot stays closer to the left foot. This stretch also gets the lower back and the iliotibial band on the outside of the leg.

A stretch for the butt:

1. Starts with the athlete on her back. The legs are out straight.
2. The massager raises the left leg up to 90 degrees with the leg bent at the knee (see illustration on page 35).
3. The knee is turned to the outside and the foot inside.
4. The massager presses the leg up and into the chest with the leg in this manner. Hold the stretch for at least 10 seconds and then repeat on the other side.

One other great stretch is for the outside of the shoulder.

1. Stand straight up with the feet shoulder-width apart.
2. The athlete brings the right arm straight across the body to the left.
3. The left arm hooks the right arm above the right elbow with the front of the left elbow (see illustration on page 55).
4. The massager, who is behind the athlete, pulls the right arm in to the body and away from the right side. Hold the stretch for at least 10 seconds and repeat on the other side.

A golfer will massage the areas that he must be careful not to injure: forearm, wrist, shoulder, and low back. Smoothing, swinging the arms in circles, and twisting the body are great to do before each stroke.

Football

Football is a collision sport. It is fast. The athletes are fast and heavy. This mix makes for a ferocious sport. A football player must be in top shape to play this game. The athlete must also be able to survive the progressively colder season with the minimum of injuries. This makes the week between games extremely important for the athlete and team. The athletes must heal, practice, and prepare for the next opponents. Football players can have just about any injury. They can break bones, tear muscles, have sprains, strains, bruises, scrapes, cuts, concussions, and more. The massager must deal with the soft-tissue injuries. The areas that need attention are the neck, shoulders, back, low back, quads, hamstrings, and ankles.

The massager will pay attention to the athlete's particular position when doing the pre-event sports massage. The position of the player and the role of the player will affect the massage. A quarterback will massage shoulders, arms, trunk, and low back. A running back will massage and stretch his legs, low back, shoulders, and forearms. Linemen will massage and stretch the legs, back, low back, trunk, and shoulders. Receivers and defensive backs massage and stretch their legs, back, low back, and shoulders.

Neck rolls and movements are done with the athlete standing or sitting on a chair. This is shown in the pre-event self massage football section. The massager can stretch the neck at all the end ranges of motion. The massager will stretch the head forward, backward, twist to the right and left, drop to the right and left, and to the front, left, and right angles. The massager can also massage the traps, shoulders, and the upper back while the athlete is in the sitting position (see the partner maintenance chapter on the shoulder).

Hockey

Hockey players have to worry about bodies, sticks, a hard puck, immovable walls, and the hard ice. They can get injuries from collisions with these objects. The hockey player has to pay special attention to the low back, hips, groin, shoulders, and legs. Goalies will massage and stretch the groin for the flexibility to get down and cover the ice in front of the net. The massager must take into account that hockey players usually hold the sticks on one side, so the opposite traps and shoulders are raised higher.

The massager will stretch the groin.

1. The athlete is sitting on the ground. The legs are bent with the feet together in the center.

2. The athlete grabs the feet.

<u>3.</u> The massager, who is behind the athlete, presses down on the knees to stretch the groin. Hold the stretch for at least 10 seconds and release.

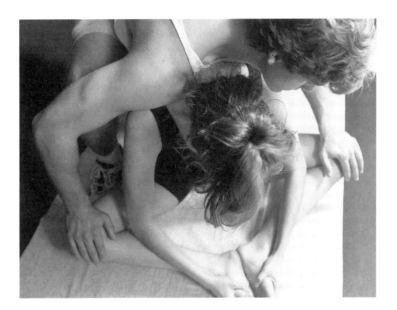

To stretch the lower back:

1. The athlete is sitting down with the legs straight and out to the sides.

2. The athlete turns the upper body to the right slightly and lowers the upper body to the left knee. Think of reaching out to the left foot instead of down to the knee.

3. The massager, who is behind the athlete, presses the left hand into the right lower back toward the left knee. The right hand of the massager presses the right leg into the ground. This stretch will stretch the right lower back (quadratus lumborum muscle). Hold the stretch for at least 10 seconds and repeat on the other side.

The athlete will do extra massage to the low back, hips, shoulders, and legs.

Martial Arts

Martial artists, like dancers, use their entire body. They will get injuries from the extreme range of motion of some of the movements. A martial artist's body must be very warm and flexible to avoid injuries. This does not take away from the fact that martial arts is a contact sport. These athletes will get injured from trauma. A martial artist will get the entire body. Each style has a different emphasis and must be taken into account: judo has throwing, so the low back and twisting will be a focus of the pre-event sports massage; tae kwon do emphasizes the legs, so the legs and lower back will be the focus. Work the areas that are highlighted. Another way to find these areas is to take a few classes and find where you feel the stress of the workouts the next few days after the practice. The areas that are sore are the focus areas.

A stretch for the back and shoulders:

1. Start with the athlete standing with the feet shoulder-width apart.
2. The arms are over the head. The hands are crossed so the right hand is on the left side and the left is on the right side.
3. The palms are facing each other, and the fingers are interlaced.
4. Breathe in, and breathe out as you lean the upper body to the left. Hold the stretch for at least 10 seconds (see illustration on page 71).
5. The massager, who is behind the athlete, pulls the raised arm away from the body and pushes the trunk down with the other arm.
6. Come back to neutral: the starting point. Breathe in, and breathe out as you repeat the stretch to the right.

Gymnastics

Gymnasts must worry about all types of injuries to the entire body. These athletes can hold their upper body up with the shoulders out to the side as in the iron cross. They catapult in the air on tumbling techniques. In general, the ankles, foot, shin, low back, shoulder, elbow, and wrist are focus areas for injuries. Because of this, gymnasts must massage the entire body. If the athlete is only doing one or two events, the events they are doing will affect the massage. For a floor routine, balance beam, and vault, the athlete will focus the massage more on the body below the chest, even though the shoulders and arms are massaged. The uneven bar, rings, and parallel bars has the athlete focus on massaging the shoulders and arms, even though the legs and back are massaged. Gymnastics events are usually shorter then most dances, but they are extremely explosive, so a gymnast should get extra massage to get the body primed for that short time period. The ankle is an important area for landing, so range-of-motion techniques are great here.

Skiing

Skiers must be careful of injuries to the hand, wrist, shoulder, low back, hips, and knees. A skier must be aware of the terrain and the elements they are doing their event in. Be careful of frostbite. Downhill skiers will massage their legs and lower back. The thighs and hips are very important in staying low and getting off that outside ski. Slalom racers should also get their arms and shoulders to help take the blow from the breakaway poles. Nordic or cross-country skiers will work the shoulders and back to get the areas that help when the upper body propels them.

A stretch for the lower back:

1. Start with the athlete sitting on the ground.
2. The bottom of the feet are together in the middle, with the knees out to the side. The hands are around the feet or ankle.
3. The athlete breathes out as she pulls her upper body to her feet.
4. The massager, who is behind her, slowly pushes her forward toward her toes. Hold the stretch for at least 10 seconds at the lowest point (see illustration on page 135).

A second stretch is as follows:

1. The athlete sits on a chair.
2. The right leg crosses the left leg so the knees are together and the right knee is over on the left side.
3. The massager pulls the athlete's body to the right so the trunk twists.

Hold the stretch for at least 10 seconds and repeat on the other side.

A massage stroke that a massager can do to a skier is to pat and rub the legs. She pats the legs vigorously down the outside and up the inside of the leg. After doing this cycle 5 times, the skier leans forward with the knees bent and the massager rubs (smoothes) the back and lower back with both hands.

Soccer

A soccer athlete has to worry about injuries to the legs and neck. Shinsplints, sprained ankles, hamstring pulls, and overuse foot injuries are common. In soccer, the athlete changes speeds and moves in all directions. These athletes must have good low back and leg strength and endurance. A soccer player will focus the massage on her legs and hips. A goalie, the only position where she can use her hands, will massage the shoulders and legs. A soccer player should also massage the neck and traps for all the heading of the ball that she might do.

Swimming

Swimmers need that great shoulder flexibility and endurance depending on the events or group of events they are competing in. Swimmers must worry about overuse injuries to the shoulders. Individual medley (IM) swimmers (swimmers that do all four strokes: back, breast, fly, free) need to condition and massage for all the strokes. A freestyler will work the shoulder and lats. A fly person will work the shoulders and hips. A breaststroke person will work their forearms, inner thighs, shoulders, and lats.

To stretch the chest and front shoulder:

1. The athlete stands with the feet shoulder-width apart.
2. She puts her arms behind her and leans her whole body forward away from the arms till she feels the stretch.
3. The massager pulls the arms further back and up. Hold the stretch for at least 10 seconds and repeat (see illustration on page 128).

To stretch the middle back:

1. The athlete is in a sitting or standing position.

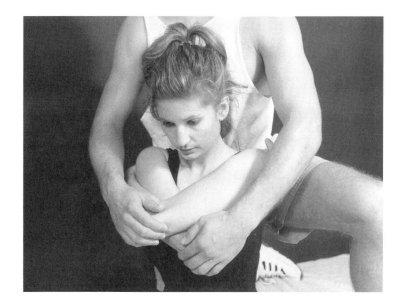

2. The athlete crosses his arms as if to give himself a hug.

3. The massager pulls the arms by the elbows away from their respective sides. Squeeze the arms so that they move away and the back arches. Feel the stretch in the middle of the back between the shoulder blades. Hold the stretch for at least 10 seconds and repeat with the other arm over the first one.

Volleyball

Volleyball players need lightning quickness and jumping ability. Volleyball players can get injuries from being hit by the ball, as in jammed finger, or from landing improperly, as in sprained ankles. The athlete needs to have great shoulder movement to spike a ball. Emphasize the legs, arms, shoulders. Work the inner and outer hips and thighs for quick lateral motion.

Weight Lifting

A weight lifter should get the entire body, but if you are breaking the body down to body parts or areas, massage those areas. An example of this would be to lift back and biceps in one workout. You will pre-event massage the back and biceps. It is also good to do some compressions or kneading to the muscle between the sets. Shaking the muscles is a must! So after the first set of bench presses, you would compress the chest, knead the deltoids and triceps or shake the area for a few seconds until your next set. Another great one is to stretch after the massage between sets, or just stretching. In the case of the bench press, stretch the chest, shoulders, and triceps, then continue with the second set. The massage will fill in the time between the sets and help you rest and rejuvenate enough to have great success in the next set. The muscles will also get the benefit of the massage. Stretch and massage the muscles that are lifting the exercise or movement.

Rowing and Kayaking

Rowing is an exercise that takes the entire body. The injuries that rowers can get are overuse injuries and muscle strains. Kayaking uses the upper body to move and the lower body usually stays stationary. Kayakers can get overuse injuries to the shoulders and stiffness in the lower back. Rowers and kayakers use the shoulders, back, chest, wrists, and upper arms a lot. These are the areas that will be emphasized. Really knead the deltoid and triceps muscles. While moving along, these athletes can take a break and shake out the tight muscle areas like weight lifters. Twisting movements for the torso are great to loosen and warm this vital area. Also, one may use the cramp techniques described in the Chapter 8.

The massager and athlete must work as a team. The massager helps to warm the athlete up. The massager also helps the athlete get more out of a stretch by increasing the range of motion of the stretch and decreasing the effort that an athlete has to expend doing these stretches. If the athlete is injured, the massager will spend extra time warming that area with massage. Do not do deep tissue work at the injury site, just extra massage.

SEVEN

Post-Event Partner Massage

The purpose of the post-event sports massage is to rejuvenate the body to help speed its healing and to cool down the athlete after the event. Unlike the pre-event, post-event partner massage starts with the athlete on his back. The front half of the body is massaged and then the back side. The ends of the strokes in post-event are a bit slower, sometimes deeper, and more rhythmic than in pre-event massage. Start the massage with medium to light depth and pace, then massage the area with slower and deeper strokes. Use a lot of compressions with a twisting motion. Look for any areas where the athlete may have developed tension or strain. Work the tension and cramps with massage and stretching, but do not do deep tissue work. Be careful to avoid any injuries that may have happened during the particular event.

Sports-specific post-event partner massages are on pages 156–172.

Chest

1. The athlete is on his back. His legs are out straight. His arms are on the ground and out to the side 45 degrees. The palms are up.
2. The massager is above the head and shoulders facing the feet.

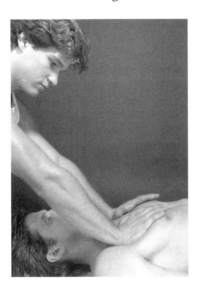

_3._ Place the heels of your hands on the top of the chest on each side. *On women do not press into the breast tissue.*

4. Compress the chest by "walking" the hands on the chest muscles. Put pressure onto the right hand, and as you are releasing the pressure, press into the left hand. It is easier to do this by moving your body over the hand that is applying the pressure. Compress in lines and circles. Hold some of the compressions and do alternating circles. Do not work on the sternum, the bone in the middle of the chest. Compress the entire chest area at least 3 times. The pace and depth is medium.

5. Finish massaging the chest by applying a deep, slow shake to the muscles.

Shoulders

1. The athlete is on her back in the same position as above.
2. The massager is above the head, also in the same position as above.
3. Grab the outside of each shoulder with your hands. Knead the shoulders with your hands. Move the hands in circles and get the front, bottom, side, and back of this shoulder muscle.
4. After at least 3 times, stop the kneading and smooth the shoulders in long, slow circles.
5. Grab the right hand in your right hand. Your left hand is on top of the right shoulder.
6. Pull the right shoulder down and away from the neck. Hold the stretch for at least 10 seconds.

7. Move back to the starting position and stand up.
8. Grab the hands in your hands and lift up the upper body off the ground 1–3 inches. Hold the athlete's hands and let her feel the stretch in the shoulders and back. Lean your body to one side while holding her hands. If you lean to the left, the left arm becomes loose (see illustration on page 117).
9. Shake out the loose arm in slow circles. Do 3 circles in each direction. Repeat on the other shoulder.
10. After doing the range of motion on the other shoulder, lower the athlete back to the ground.
11. Move just below her hips, stand over her, and face her head.
12. Grab her hands again and raise her body off the ground 1–5 inches. Vary the height of the lift to stretch different parts of her back. The massager can also grab the hands on the other side of her body to get a different and enjoyable stretch.
13. After finishing the stretches and lowering her to the ground, keep her hands in yours and the arms in the air.
14. Shake the right arm in slow motions for at least 10 seconds.
15. Stop and repeat the shaking of the shoulder on the other side for the same time.
16. Finish the chest and shoulders by lowering her arms to the ground.

Arms and Hands

1. The athlete is on her back and in the same position as above.
2. The massager is by the hips, facing the athlete's head.
3. With your right hand, grab the right hand as if you were giving a handshake. With the left hand, knead the whole deltoid muscle (shoulder muscle) (see illustration on page 115).
4. Knead the area for at least 10 seconds.
5. Place the heel of your left hand on the biceps.
6. Compress the biceps from the deltoid to the front elbow. Do this at least 3 times.
7. Move down to the outside of the elbow.
8. Her right palm is now down on the ground.

9. Compress the outside forearm from the elbow to the wrist. Compress down and up 3 times.

10. Stop and move to the inside of the elbow.

11. Her right palm is now up.

12. Compress the inside forearm from the elbow to the wrist. Compress down and up 3 times. In all of these strokes, the pace and depth is medium.

13. Move to the right hand of the athlete.

14. Her palm is up in your left hand as you massage the hand on the ground.

15. Compress around the palm of the hand with your right loose fist at least 4 times.

16. Finish the area by shaking them vigorously.

Neck Stretch

1. The athlete is on his back with the arms relaxed by his side and his legs straight out.

2. The massager is above the athlete's head, facing the feet.

3. Cross both hands to the opposite shoulder on the front of the shoulder.

4. Ask the athlete to take a deep breath in and to breathe all the way out slowly. As the athlete breathes out, the massager lifts the head slowly so the chin of the athlete moves to touch the chest. If the athlete is too tight or the stretch is uncomfortable, hold at a point where he comfortably feels the stretch. Hold the stretch at its greatest point for at least 10 seconds. Remind the athlete to continue to breathe.

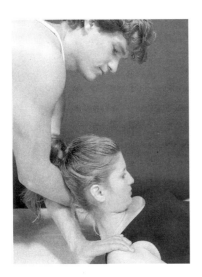

5. Release the stretch by having the athlete take another deep breath in and out. The massager lowers the head slowly as he breathes out.

6. With the head on the ground, angle yourself to the athlete's left shoulder.

7. Place your right hand on the left side of the athlete's head above the ear and the left hand on the left shoulder.

8. Have the athlete breathe in again. Stretch the head to the right shoulder as he breathes out.

Hold the stretch at its furthest comfortable point for at least 10 seconds.

9. Release the head to neutral as above, with the breath.
10. Stretch the other side.
11. Continue the process of having the athlete breathe as you stretch the neck at angles between the first one to the front and those to the sides.
12. Do the same sequence for stretching the neck to each side in rotations, left and right. To stretch the neck to the left, place your right hand on the left back of the head and the left hand on the right front side of the head.

Back Stretch

1. The athlete is on her back. The legs are out straight and the arms are relaxed by her side.
2. The massager is standing over her head, facing her feet.
3. Squat down and grab the athlete's wrists, your left in her right and your right in her left.
4. Straighten your legs as you pull on her arms to lift her upper body off the ground. Her upper body makes an angle of 10 to 50 degrees to the ground. The athlete will feel the stretch in her back as she hangs from your arms. Hold the stretch for at least 10 seconds (see illustration on page 117).
5. Lower the athlete if your hands slip on her wrists. This is overcome by having her grab and continue to hold your wrists. When she lets go, you have less to hold as her wrist tendons loosen and she slips.
6. Also do the back stretch by pulling one side of her body up higher than the other. Lower that upper side so that each is equal and then do the other side by raising it higher. You can do this by shifting your body from one side (the opposite one that you want to raise) to the other.
7. Lower her upper body to the ground slowly so the tension in her shoulders released. Continue to hold her wrists.
8. Move her arms in small, slow circles (both directions). Repeat the circles at least 3 times to relax the shoulder musculature that helped to hold her up.
9. Move to her hips.
10. Grab the opposite lower back with your hands.

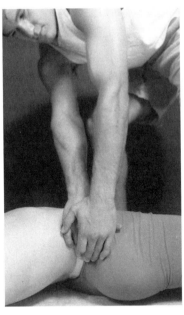

11. Pull the back by the hip up off the floor in a twisting motion. Hold the stretch for at least 10 seconds. Repeat on the other side.

12. Finish by placing her arms at her sides on the ground.

Groin

1. The athlete is on her back. The legs are out straight and the arms are at her side.

2. The massager is on the athlete's right side, by the knees.

3. Bring the right leg up and out so the knee is off the ground to the outside and the sole of her foot is by the other knee.

4. Place one or both of your legs by your knee underneath her knee to stabilize her leg.

5. Compress the inside of her leg with the heel of your right hand. The left hand holds the leg by the knee. The pace and depth are medium. Start with light pressure to get the gracilis muscle to loosen and then get deeper into the other adductor muscles. Compress up and down to the hip at least 3 times. Avoid the groin and front of the hip where the leg meets the hip, which are areas of sensitive nerves and blood vessels (see illustration on page 118).

6. Stop and then stretch the groin muscles by moving your legs, placing your right hand on her left hip, the left hand on her knee, and gently pressing the knee down to the ground. Avoid pressing with the right hand into the bony points of the hip, which hurts.

7. Finish the area by shaking the area vigorously to energize it.

Front Upper Leg

1. The athlete is on his back with the legs out straight and the arms relaxed.

2. The massager is kneeling by the athlete's right leg, with the left hand on the outside upper leg and the right hand by the knee.

3. Compress with the heel of your left hand down the outside of the thigh in straight lines from hip to knee. Hold some of the compressions. Press the held compressions into the muscles and down to stretch the tissues out. Do the compressions on the upper leg at least 3 times (see illustration on page 119).
4. Then move to the top of the thigh and the outside of the thigh.
5. Compress each line at least 3 times. Press the inside of the right knee with your right hand to have the outside of the thigh showing to the heel of your left hand.
6. After getting the outside and top of the front thigh, hold the left hand just below the hip and compress the inside of the thigh with the left heel of your hand. Get the area from the knee to the hip. The line moves slightly to the outside or top of the thigh as the left hand compresses up the front thigh. Do this at least 3 times.
7. Stop and face your body to the other front thigh.
8. Knead the front right thigh with both hands from knee to hip and inside to outside at least 3 times.
9. Finish the massage on the front thigh by shaking the thigh with both hands, the right hand on the inside and the left hand on the outside. The leg can slightly rotate from side to side, which will help release the hip muscles.

Hamstring Stretch

1. The athlete is on her back. The legs are out straight and the arms are relaxed by her side.
2. The massager is on the athlete's right side by the lower leg. The massager is facing her head.
3. Grab the right ankle above the back heel with the right hand and hold above the knee with the left to keep the entire leg straight.
4. Lift the right leg up toward the upper body to stretch the hamstring muscles. Hold the stretch at its highest point for at least 10 seconds. It is better to hold the stretch here for much longer. This muscle, if tight, can cause a lot of lower back pain! The stretch can happen at many ranges of motion. For very tight people, the leg only has to be raised a

few inches off the ground. For people who are flexible, the leg has to be raised past the 90 degree mark (straight up). Be careful to keep the leg straight or the hamstring will not be stretched as much. Make sure that the other leg stays on the ground or it will loosen the stretch. Look at the same hip to make sure that the butt does not come off the ground. To get different sides of the hamstrings, angle the leg into or away from the body about 15 degrees at the higher points of the stretch (see illustration on page 120).

5. Release the stretch by bringing the leg down to the ground gently.

Front Lower Leg

1. The athlete is on his back. The legs are out straight and the arms are relaxed.
2. The massager is down by the feet, angled up toward the opposite shoulder.
3. The right hand holds the top of the ankle and the left hand is below the right knee on the outside of the lower leg.
4. Compress the front outside lower leg with the left hand. Hold some compressions and press the hand down to the ankle to stretch the tissues. Compress the area from the bottom of the knee to the top of the outside of the ankle (see illustration on page 121).
5. After at least 3 times, turn the foot in to the body with the right hand and compress in straight lines toward the outer part of the lower leg. Compress the area all the way out to the outside of the lower leg, just before the start of the calves.
6. The massager moves up to the hip of the athlete.
7. The massager places the right palm on the muscles of the lower outside leg below the knee.
8. Slowly let the palm of your hand slide down the outside lower leg.
9. After the compressions, grab the inside edge of the right foot with the right hand. The left hand holds the ankle and stabilizes the leg so it does not move.
10. Using the right hand, move the ankle up and down at a medium pace so the toes of the feet point to the body and then away from the body. Do this at least 3 times.

11. Stretch the ankle at the end range of motions at the top and bottom of the movements.
12. Using the hands in the same way, turn the foot in and out so the bottom of the foot turns in and out. (The foot turns in more than it turns out.) Do not do this or the next range-of-motion exercise on an athlete with a sprained ankle! Do this at least 3 times.
13. Turn the ankle in the largest circles that the foot can go with the same hand positioning. Circle both ways at least 3 times.
14. Finish the lower leg with fast light compressions on the lower leg muscles.

Feet

1. The athlete is on his back with the legs out straight and the arms relaxed.
2. The massager is at his feet and facing the other foot.
3. The massager presses the loose right fist into the bottom of the foot.
4. Do light circular compressions to the bottom of the foot.
5. Do light circular frictioning with your thumbs or fingers. Massage the area from the toes to the heel of the ankle at a medium pace.
6. Finish the foot by placing the left palm on top of the foot and the right palm on the bottom of the foot.
7. Rub the foot vigorously to warm the area.
8. Repeat on the other leg.

Back

1. The athlete is on his stomach. His head is to the side and the legs out straight. The feet are out to the side or where they are comfortable. The arms are at the sides and straight or up by the shoulders and bent at the elbow. (One or both hands can be underneath the head to cushion it.)
2. The massager moves to the right side of the body.
3. Start by rhythmically pushing the body back and forth.
4. Place your hands on the left side of the back, just across the spine by the left shoulder blade. *Do not press onto the spine!*
5. Compress the erector spinae muscles down with the heel of your left hand. The right hand can stay where it is or can move down with the other hand. It feels best if one hand holds the body while the other one does the mas-

sage. Move the hand 1–2 inches down each compression. Compress down to the top of the hip and continue back up the body. As you compress back up, move slightly to the outside of the left erector muscles. Do this 3–5 times at least. Compress at a medium pace and medium depth.

6. To stretch the lower back, the massager crosses his arms and presses the right hand on the right ribs and the left hand presses on the top of the right hip.

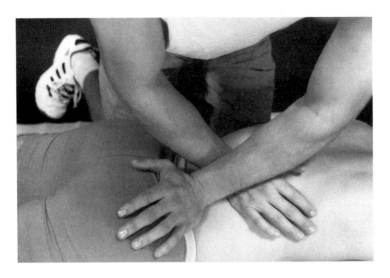

7. Lean over the arms and think of stretching the lower back.

8. End the strokes with slower and deeper pace and depth to relax and cool down the body.

9. Stop at the top by the upper shoulder blade.

10. Compress the inside of the top edge of the shoulder blade. This is the attachment of a neck muscle (levator scapula). It may be sore, so do not work it too hard. Stay at a medium to light pace and depth till you end the strokes at this area.

11. Then massage the area with slower and deeper strokes. Massage the area for at least 10 seconds.

12. Massage back down the back to just above the hips. The right hand can move down to the middle of the back.

13. Compress down into the low back muscles. Angle some of the compressions down and up into the tissue to stretch the muscles. Work for at least 10 seconds here. Compress at a slower pace than above and hold the compression into the tissue a tiny bit longer.

Shoulder Blade
1. The athlete and massager are in the same positions as above.
2. Slowly shake the athlete's body back and forth, from side to side, as you move up to the shoulder blade. Move your hands over to the right shoulder blade. It is easier to position yourself by the right hip to be angled up to her body.
3. Compress into the right shoulder blade with the right heel of your hand. Push the shoulder blade in different directions with your compressions to loosen the musculature around the shoulder blade.
4. Compress the outside angle of the shoulder blade as well as on top of the shoulder blade. Compress the area for at least 30 seconds at a medium pace and a light to medium depth.

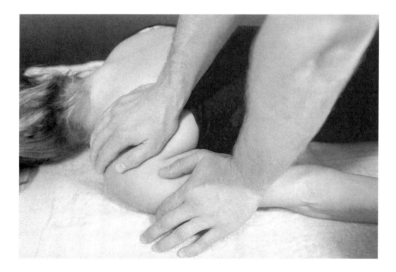

5. Shake the shoulder blade with the right hand.
6. Smooth the middle of the back with long, slow strokes. The stroke looks like the massager is wiping off the back or applying a strip down both sides of the spine.
7. Move your body to the left side and repeat the back and shoulder blade massages.

Neck

1. The athlete is on his stomach.
2. The massager is on either side of the body by the shoulder blade area and angled to the head.
3. With one hand, grab the neck as one would grab the nape of the neck of a cat or dog.
4. Slowly pull and let your fingers slide up toward you. Slowly increase the kneading (the stroke that you are doing) of the neck muscle this way from the bottom of the head to the base of the neck. Take about 30 seconds to massage the neck at a light depth.
5. End the stroke slowly and a little deeper to relax the athlete.
6. Press the tips of the fingers into the back of the neck.
7. Circular friction the back of the neck from the bottom of the head to the top of the back in small, slow circles. The pressure is light.
8. Repeat 6 and 7 on the other side of the neck.
9. Repeat the neck and shoulder on the other side.

Butt

1. Move your body to the hips on the left side.
2. Compress into the butt with your fists. Compress in horizontal lines and around as you get the entire butt area from the middle of their body out to the hip area. Work on the top part of the butt by the lower back. This is a major area for dancers or other athletes who stand on one leg or move from side to side. Compress for at least 30 seconds. Work at a medium pace and depth (see illustration on page 190).
3. Press in with the palm and shake the muscles out at a fast pace.
4. Finish by pressing down just below the base of the spine between the left and right butt cheeks (the sacrum bone). Do this by standing over them, facing the upper body, one leg on each side, and the palms of the hands pressing the sacrum down and to the lower legs. Hold the pressure for at least 10 seconds.

Hamstrings

1. The athlete is still on her stomach.

2. The massager is on her left side between the knee and hip.
3. Place the heel of the left hand into the back thigh area. The right hand is down by the knee, either on the hamstring or just below the knee on the calf muscles (see top illustration on page 111).
4. Compress with the heel of your hand down the middle back thigh from the bottom of the butt to the top of the knee. Stay with the compressions for a longer time if the weather is cold. Massage this area at least 3 times at a medium pace and depth.
5. Place the right heel of the hand (or a loose fist) on the inside of the left hamstring right below the butt. The left hand is down by the bottom of the hamstrings or on the top of the calf muscles. Compress down the inner hamstring from this starting point to the top of the inner knee. Move the hand slightly down each compression (1–2 inches). Compress at a medium pace and depth at least 3 times.
6. After this, turn your body toward the leg.
7. Knead the entire hamstring area with both hands. Emphasize the upper and middle hamstrings.
8. Finish by shaking the entire area from the butt to the knee.

Iliotibial Band

1. The athlete is on her stomach.
2. The massager is on her left side by the knee, angled toward the right shoulder.
3. Have the athlete bring the left knee up to the left side so the athlete's outside thigh is showing. *Only do this massage work if the athlete is comfortable, with no pain in the hip or knee.*
4. The massager's left hand is holding her left knee to the ground. The right palm heel of the hand compresses the middle of the outside of the thigh from the hip down to just above the knee. Compress down and up the thigh at a medium pace and depth (lighten the depth if the massage is painful) at least 3 times (see bottom illustration on page 111).
5. Finish by smoothing down the thigh 2–3 times at a light and fast pace and depth.
6. Bring the leg back to a straight position so the hamstrings are again showing.

Quad Stretch
1. The athlete is still on his stomach.
2. The massager is down between the left knee and the left hip.
3. With the right hand, grab the front of the left ankle.
4. Bend the lower leg so the heel of the left foot goes to the butt.
5. Move the leg in slowly till the athlete feels the stretch in the front of the left thigh. The heel of the foot may be pressed into the butt. Hold the stretch for at least 10 seconds. Sometimes it is great to hold the stretch for a few minutes so the athlete can really feel the stretch.
6. Release the stretch slowly and return the foot to the floor.
7. Repeat the stretch if needed.

Hip Flexor Stretch
1. The athlete and the massager are in the same position as above.
2. The massager is kneeling on one leg, the left further forward than the right.
3. Bend the athlete's left knee to decrease the angle between the foot and the butt with the right hand.
4. Place her left foot on the front of your right shoulder.
5. Grab the inside left knee with the right hand (see top illustration on page 113).
6. The left hand presses into the middle of her left butt.
7. Lift the left knee up off the ground by leaning forward to the left leg. The knee may go about 0–4 inches up off the ground depending on her flexibility. To keep the lower back from arching the massager tells the athlete to contract her abdominal muscles. Hold the stretch for at least 10 seconds. Hold the stretch longer if this area is tight or the athlete has lower back problems.
8. Release the stretch slowly and bring the knee to the ground.
9. Keeping your hold on the foot, lift the leg off the ground slightly to drop the leg to the ground. Raise and drop the leg at a fast pace so the leg hits the ground gently. This action lets the ground tapot the front of the thigh. Do this for at least 10 seconds.
10. Stop the tapotment and lower the foot to the ground.

Calves

1. The athlete is still on his back.
2. The massager is down between the left knee and the left foot.
3. Place the right heel of your hand on the inside left calf muscle just below the knee. The left hand is immobile on the outside of the top left knee (see bottom illustration on page 113).
4. Compress with the heel of the hand or a loose fist down to above the left heel of the foot. Make sure that the athlete's foot is comfortable. Move up and down this area 3 times with constantly deeper pressure till you get to a medium depth. The pace is also medium throughout.
5. Repeat the compressions on the outside of the calves.
6. Keep the right hand down by the ankle as the left hand compresses the area from below the knee to the ankle.
7. After doing the compressions 3 times, knead the area with both hands. Especially get the top three-quarters of the lower leg.
8. Finish by smoothing the entire lower leg slowly.

Tibialis Anterior Stretch

1. The athlete is on her back with her legs straight out.
2. The massager is down by the right foot.
3. Grab the right foot with your right hand and the top of the back of the ankle with your left hand.

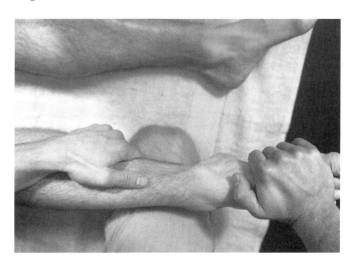

4. Put the front ankle on your kneeling left knee.

5. Pull the foot so the toes go away from the body (as in pointing; plantar flexion). Make sure that the athlete feels the stretch on the front of the lower leg. Hold the stretch for at least 10 seconds.

6. Finish the stretch by releasing and slowly lowering the foot and leg to the ground.

Feet

1. The athlete is on his stomach with the legs out straight. His shoes are off.

2. The massager is facing his head while being below his feet. Place your fists into the bottoms of the feet.

3. Compress the bottoms of the feet with the fists (knuckle area). Compress the area from the heel to the toes. The pressure here is from medium to deep and the pace is medium (see illustration on page 114).

4. Press and hold the soft, loose fist at the bottom of the foot just in front of the ankle. Finish the foot by smoothing the entire area slowly.

5. Get the entire lower, right extremity from the butt to the feet. Then flip the athlete over onto her back.

SPORTS-SPECIFIC POST-EVENT PARTNER MASSAGE
Running, Hiking, Jogging

In any type of running, hiking, or jogging event—the hurdles, sprints, marathons, or jogging—the massager will spend most of the time on the legs, butt, abs, and lower back. He will stretch the same areas: legs, butt, and trunk (all around the midsection). If the event is high intensity running or hiking, as in sprinting, hurdles, or heavy backpacking, the massager will massage and stretch the shoulder, chest, and upper back. The massager does ankle range of motions: circle the ankle in the largest circles, point the toes up and down, turn ankle in and out, and squeeze the toes in and spread them out. The athlete can do circular compressions, smoothing, or shaking and jostling to the abs, low back, butt, quads, hamstrings, calves, and front lower leg.

The massager should stretch the hips (similar to a lunge stretch), groin, calf, and soleus, and do ankle and hip range of motions. The massager should do smoothing and shaking the body from below the ribs. The strokes are slow and rhythmic.

The partner lunge stretch:

1. Start out with the athlete on his back with the arms relaxed.
2. The massager bends the left leg at the knee, then lifts the leg up and pushes the knee toward the chest.
3. The end position has the athlete's knee as close to the chest as possible. The right leg does not come off the ground (see top illustration on page 123).
4. The massager ends the stretch by lowering the leg back to the ground.

Instead of doing the stretch, the massager can just lift the leg up to the chest and lower it back done in fluid motions. Do the top of the range of motion in angles away and across the body. The massager can also keep the leg off the ground and circle the leg so the hip is moved in circles. This is a great hip range-of-motion technique.

The groin stretch:

1. The athlete is on her back.
2. The massager brings the right leg out to the left side as far as it will go.
3. The massager's left leg stabilizes the right leg of the athlete so that it does not cross over to the left (see bottom illustration on page 123).

The calf stretch is best done by the athlete. Therefore, the athlete will do the same stretch as in the pre-event self massage chapter (see bottom illustration on page 46). The soleus stretch is the same, but the knee of the stretched leg is bent to get the muscle underneath (see illustration on page 47). It is also important to hold the legs raised above the body while the athlete is on his back. This will let gravity bring the blood back to the body so the body does not have to do the work.

Tennis and Racquetball

The massager will spend most of his time on the shoulder, forearms, adductors, hamstrings, and calves of the athlete. He will also stretch these areas. The massager can do circular compressions, smoothing, and shaking and jostling to the legs, trunk, and shoulders after a match or practice. The massager massages the forearm, arm, and shoulder that the tennis player uses with slow and rhythmic strokes. Compressions and some light holding of the muscle tissue is excellent. The top and outside of the butt is also a great area to massage in this pattern.

1. To stretch the chest, the athlete is sitting on a chair or sitting on the ground with the legs crossed in front of him.

2. The athlete raises his arms to shoulder height to the sides and bend the elbow so the arms look like goal posts.

3. The massager, who is behind the athlete, grabs the front side of the elbows. The massager pulls the arms to the back and the athlete feels the stretch in the chest.

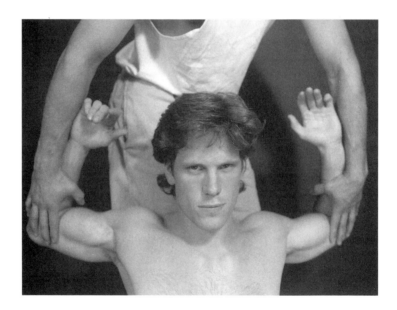

Another great stretch for these athletes is the hip and groin stretch, described in the running section.

The partner stretch for the iliotibial band:

1. Start with the athlete on her back with the legs out straight.

2. The massager brings the athlete's right foot across the left leg by the knee.

3. The massager places his left hand on her right hip and the right hand goes to the outside of the right knee (see illustration on page 125).

4. Holding the leg down with the left hand, the massager pushes the leg across the body and down to the left side. The leg will not move too far. Hold the stretch for at least 10 seconds and repeat on the other side.

The massager can also knead the shoulders with his hands. Other great areas to massage are the lower back, trunk (twisting stretches), shoulder range of motions, and wrist shaking.

Baseball

The athletes should massage the neck, traps, shoulders, upper arms, elbows, forearms, wrists, and hands. The lower back and hamstrings should also be emphasized in the massage. The massager should move the shoulders in all its movements and ranges of motion. A pitcher will stretch out the arm.

The triceps stretch, shown in the pre-event self massage general workout, is great. Begin as for the self massage:

1. Reach and place the left hand on the top of the left shoulder.
2. Place the right hand on the left elbow.
3. Push the left arm up to the ceiling while keeping the left hand in contact with the shoulder. Do not arch the back (see top illustration on page 56).
4. The massager can grab the raised elbow to help stretch the arm more.
5. The athlete then brings both arms to the back and clasps the hands.
6. The massager will then raise the arms to the back. Hold the stretch at its highest point for at least 10 seconds, release, and repeat. This stretch stretches the front of the shoulder and the chest muscles.

The massager then does the infraspinatus stretches.

1. The athlete is standing or sitting.
2. The athlete puts the back of his hand on his lower back (same side) (see middle illustration on page 56).
3. The massager grabs the arm at the elbow and pulls the arm forward so the athlete feels the stretch on the back of the shoulder blade.
4. The massager stretches the subscapularis muscle by having the right arm by the athlete's right side. The elbow of the right arm is bent to a 90-degree angle.

5. The massager grabs the right hand in his right hand and uses his left hand to hold the athlete's elbow in at the side of the body.

6. The massager then pulls the arm away from the front of the body while keeping the elbow at his side. Hold the stretch for at least 10 seconds and then repeat.

A catcher will also stretch out his quads, hamstrings, and lower back. The first baseman will stretch the arms and legs with particular attention to the hamstrings and groin to increase the catching stretch. The side that a baseball player uses will get the most attention in stretching and massage, but, as for any training, the other side must get worked on.

Another great stretch for baseball players is for the chest and front shoulders.

1. The athlete is sitting on the ground or a chair.

2. The massager is behind the athlete.

3. The athlete has his hands interlaced behind his head.

4. The massager grabs the elbows and pulls them back. Hold the stretch for at least 10 seconds and repeat (see illustration on page 158).

Basketball

The massager will massage the lower back, quads, hamstrings, calves, groin, feet, shoulders, and forearms. Basketball players need to spend more time in a stretch and massaging the area that is stretched because of the large number of games that they play. The massager can do the stretches described in the running section. The massager can hold the stretches and knead or compress the stretched muscles. Kneading and compressing are repeated after each stretch of the lower body and any stretch to one side of the upper body.

To stretch the shoulder:

1. First, the athlete is on his knees facing the massager.

2. The athlete bends her upper body forward (see illustration on page 62).

3. The massager grabs the athlete's hands and raises the arms above her head slowly. This stretches the lats, chest, and lower part of the shoulder capsule.

A second stretch for the shoulder:

1. The athlete sits on the ground with her legs out straight and together.
2. She then places her arms behind her body and the massager grabs the arms and pulls them up behind her to stretch the chest and shoulder (see illustration on page 128).

A stretch for the back:

1. Start with the athlete sitting on the ground with the knees to the outside and the feet together in the middle.
2. The athlete grabs his feet and drops his head.
3. The massager, behind the athlete, pushes the upper body of the athlete slowly down to his feet. Hold the stretch for at least 10 seconds (see illustration on page 135).

To stretch the butt:

1. The athlete starts out lying on his back.
2. The massager, kneeling on the right side of the athlete, brings the athlete's right knee to his chest.
3. The massager turns the hip in so the right foot moves to the left side. The side of the right thigh is now facing the athlete. The stretch is felt in the butt and may be felt in the iliotibial band on the side of the thigh. Hold the stretch for at least 10 seconds.

Bicycling

The areas that bikers will be massaged and stretched are the thighs (quads and hamstrings), hips, lower leg (front and back), low back, shoulder, arms, wrists, and neck.

A massage technique for the lower back:

1. Start with the athlete lying on his right side.
2. The athlete's left arm and bent left leg are on the floor for support. The right leg is straight (see illustration on page 79).
3. The massager is behind the athlete and places the right palm on the outside of the lower back muscles (left erectors) in the area between the ribs and the hips.

4. With circular compressions, the massager compresses the lower back, butt, and outer thigh of the athlete.

One stretch that is great for the soleus muscle, hips, and low back:
1. The athlete lies on her back.
2. The massager, who is below the feet, brings the athlete's knees to her chest. The athlete's feet are resting on the massager (see top illustration on page 129).
3. The massager holds the stretch for the lower back, then grabs behind the head and pulls the head of the athlete into her stretch. Hold the stretch for at least 10 seconds and then repeat.

Another stretch for a biker is the partner lunge stretch, which is described in the running section (see top illustration on page 123).

A modified "bookcase" range-of-motion technique is great for the lower back:
1. Start with the athlete down on her back.
2. The knees are bent and in the air. The feet are on the ground.
3. The massager is kneeling on one leg.
4. The massager lifts the legs off the ground and places them on one leg (see bottom illustration on page 129).
5. The massager moves the legs in circles, 3–4 in each direction.

One important massage stroke for bikers is to jostle, tapot, knead, compress, shake, or smooth the quads and hamstrings slowly after the race.
1. To tapot the quads, the athlete lies on his stomach.
2. The massager grabs a foot and bends the athlete's knee 90 degrees.
3. The massager then raises the leg off the ground and bounces the leg on the ground at a fast pace. Do the tapotment off the ground for at least 30 seconds (see top illustration on page 130).
4. Stop and then bend the ankle forward to the ground and hold the stretch to the soleus muscle. Lower the leg back to the ground. Repeat on the other side (see bottom illustration on page 130).

Bowling

The massager must stretch and warm the athlete's torso. Bowling is a sport and one must prepare for bowling as such. The low back, shouldesr, hips, hamstrings, back, forearms, and wrists are also important areas.

A stretch for the low back:

1. Start with the athlete standing up with the feet shoulder-width apart and the arms at her sides.
2. She breathes out and leans to the right side.
3. She reaches over the body with the left arm to increase the stretch and to help stretch the lats (see bottom illustration on page 56).
4. The massager will pull the arm further away and down to get a deeper stretch. Hold the stretch for at least 10 seconds, take a deep breath in, and return to the starting position.
5. Repeat on the other side and then get both sides again.

To stretch the low back, spine, and outer thigh:

1. The athlete starts by sitting down on the ground. The legs are out straight.
2. The left foot is moved across the right leg and the foot is flat on the ground by the knee.
3. The athlete looks to the left side and behind her.
4. The massager presses his left hip into her back.
5. The massager grabs the left leg of the athlete and pulls it to the right. The massager also grabs the left shoulder and pulls that to the left. Hold the stretch for at least 10 seconds and repeat on the other side. The hamstrings and hips should be stretched.

Dance and Aerobics

The whole body is worked on, and the emphasis of the post-event sports massage will depend on the particular dance that will be done. The entire body should be massaged from the neck down: neck, shoulders, back, low back, hips, abdominals, quads, hamstrings, groin, calves, shins, and feet. Really pump with compression, and twist and pull the muscles with kneading to loosen and move the fluids in the muscles after a dance. For stretches, dancers should hold the stretches for a long time: 1–5 minutes. A dancer usually has an established routine of stretches. In addition to your stretches, add circular compressions, jostling, shaking, and smoothing to the muscle that is being stretched before and after the stretch.

Golf

A golfer will massage and stretch the lower back, trunk, hips, shoulders, and insides of the forearms to get the wrist muscles. Do pelvic tilts after a day of golf:

1. Lie on your back. The hips and knees are bent with the knees in the air and the feet on the ground.
2. Tilt the pelvis backward so the low back presses into the ground.
3. Relax and tilt the pelvis forward so the lower back comes off the ground slightly.
4. Repeat the rocking motion.
5. The massager can help the rocking by kneeling on the right side of the athlete by the hips. The athlete's legs are raised so the feet are on the massager's legs.
6. The massager places the hands behind and underneath the athlete's lower back.
7. The massager now rocks along with the athlete to do the pelvic tilts.

Great stretches for golfers are the partner lunge stretch (shown in the running section—see illustration on page 123), the modified "bookcase" (in the bicycling section—see illustration on page 129), and the following one for the lower back:

1. The athlete lies on his back. The legs are out straight and the arms are at his side.
2. The athlete bends the right leg at the hip and knee so the knee is pointing straight up from the hip to the sky (see top illustration on page 123).
3. The massager presses the right knee down over to the left side so the right leg goes to the ground on the left side.
4. The massager holds the right shoulder of the athlete to the ground with her left hand. The back will now rise off the ground, but try to keep it

flat. Hold the stretch for at least 10 seconds and then return to the starting position and repeat on the other side.

Another way to do this stretch is:
1. Lie flat. Bend the right leg only at the hip (not at the knee), and keep the right leg straight as you lower it over the left leg to the ground (see illustration on page 133).
2. The leg may not make it to the ground or you will have to lower the leg so the foot stays closer to the left foot. This stretch also gets the lower back and the iliotibial band on the outside of the leg.

A stretch for the butt:
1. Start with the athlete on her back. The legs are out straight.
2. The massager raises the right leg up to 90 degrees with the leg bent at the knee. The knee is turned to the outside and the foot inside (see illustration on page 44).
3. The massager presses the leg up and into the chest with the leg in this manner. Hold the stretch for at least 10 seconds and then repeat on the other side.

One other great stretch is for the outside of the shoulder:
1. Stand straight up with the feet shoulder-width apart.
2. The athlete brings the right arm straight across the body to the left.
3. The left arm hooks the right arm above the right elbow with the front of the left elbow (see illustration on page 55).
4. The massager, who is behind the athlete, pulls the right arm in to the body and away from the right side. Hold the stretch for at least 10 seconds and repeat on the other side.

A golfer will massage the areas that he must be careful not to injure: forearms, wrists, shoulders, and low back. Smoothing, swinging the arms in circles, and twisting of the body are all great to do before each stroke.

Football

After the game, the athletes must heal, practice, and prepare for the next opponents. Football players can have just about any injury. They can break bones, tear muscles, have sprains, strains, bruises, scrapes, cuts, concussions, and more. The massager must deal with the soft-tissue injuries. The areas that need attention are the neck, shoulders, back, low back, quads, hamstrings, and ankles.

The massager will pay attention to the athlete's particular position when doing the post-event sports massage. The position of the player and the role of the player will affect the massage. A quarterback will massage shoulders, arms, trunk, and low back. A running back will massage and stretch his legs, low back, shoulders, and forearms. Linemen will massage and stretch the legs, back, low back, trunk, and shoulders. Receivers and defensive backs massage and stretch their legs, back, low back, and shoulders. The massager will massage the hamstrings with lots of compressions to pump the fluids out and into them. Massage the traps and shoulders while the athlete is sitting.

Have the athlete do neck rolls and stretch the quads, hamstrings, low back, and calves.

Hockey

The hockey player has to pay special attention to the low back, hips, groin, shoulders, and legs. Goalies will massage and stretch the groin for the flexibility to get down and cover the ice in front of the net. The massager must take into account that hockey players usually hold the sticks on one side, so the opposite traps and shoulders are raised higher. Do compressions to the shoulders and lower back, and knead the neck and quads with slow, rhythmic strokes for a long period of time.

Martial Arts

A martial artist will get the entire body massaged. Each style has a different emphasis and must be taken into account: judo has throwing, so the low back and twisting will be a focus of the post-event sports massage; tae kwon do emphasizes the legs, so the legs and lower back will be the focus. Work the areas that are highlighted. Another way to find these areas is to take a few classes and find where you feel the stress of the workouts the next few days after the practice. The areas that are sore are the focus areas.

A stretch for the back and shoulders:

1. Start with the athlete standing with the feet shoulder-width apart. The arms are over the head.
2. The hands are crossed so the right hand is on the left side and the left is on the right side. The palms are facing each other. The fingers are interlaced.
3. Breathe in, and breathe out as you lean the upper body to the left. Hold the stretch for at least 10 seconds. Come back to neutral: the starting point. Breathe in, and breathe out as you repeat the stretch to the right (see illustration on page 71).

Gymnastics

Gymnasts must massage the entire body. If the athlete is only doing one or two events, the events they are doing will affect the massage. For a floor routine, balance beam, and vault, the athlete will focus the massage more on the body below the chest, even though the shoulders and arms are massaged. The uneven bar, rings, and parallel bars has the athlete focus on massaging the shoulders and arms, even though the legs and back are massaged. Gymnastics events are usually shorter than most dances, but are extremely explosive, so a gymnast should get extra massage to get the body primed for that short time period.

The massager will spend lots of time on the area that the athlete just used. The shoulders, upper back, chest, and arms would be the focus in the rings event. The rest of the body might then just be smoothed and shaken. The ankle is an important area for landing, so range-of-motion techniques are great here.

Skiing

Downhill skiers will massage their legs and lower back. The thighs and hips are very important in staying low and getting off that outside ski. Slalom racers should also get their arms and shoulders to help take the blow from the breakaway poles. Nordic or cross-country skiers will work the shoulder and back to get the areas that help when the upper body propels them.

A stretch for the lower back:

1. Start with the athlete sitting on the ground. The sides of the feet are together in the middle, the legs straight.

2. The massager is behind the athlete.

3. The athlete breathes out as she pulls her upper body over her legs to her feet.

4. The massager pushes the upper body of the athlete further to the feet. Hold the stretch for at least 10 seconds at the lowest point.

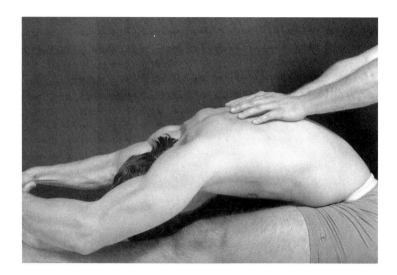

This stretch can be modified by having the athlete spread the legs as wide as they go. The massager then pushes the upper body forward to the ground in between the legs as far away from the body as possible.

A second stretch is as follows:

1. The athlete sits on a chair.

2. The right leg crosses the left leg with the right foot over the knee. The right knee is pointing to the right side.

3. The athlete pushes the right knee down to the ground and feels the stretch in the butt. Hold the stretch for at least 10 seconds and repeat on the other side.

A massage stroke that a skier can do is to pat and rub the legs. She pats the legs vigorously down the outside and up the inside of the leg. After doing this cycle 5 times, she leans forward and rubs (smoothes) the lower back with both hands on their respective side.

Soccer

A soccer player will have the massage focus on her legs and hips. A goalie, the only position where she can use her hands, will massage the shoulders and legs. A soccer player should also massage the neck (and do neck rolls) and traps for all the heading of the ball that she might do. Spend a lot of time massaging the legs with slow, rhythmic strokes to loosen the muscles.

Swimming

Individual medley (IM) swimmers (swimmers that do all four strokes: back, breast, fly, free) need to condition and massage for all the strokes. A freestyler will work the shoulder and lats. A fly person will work the shoulders and hips. A breaststroke person will work their forearms, inner thighs, shoulders, and lats.

To stretch the chest and front shoulder:

1. The athlete sits on the ground with her legs out in front of her.
2. She puts her arms behind her and leans her whole body forward away from the arms till she feel the stretch. Hold the stretch for at least 10 seconds and repeat (see illustration on page 63).

To stretch the middle back:

1. The athlete is in a sitting or standing position.
2. The athlete crosses his arms as if to give himself a hug.
3. The massager, who is behind the athlete, squeezes the arms so that they move away and the back arches. Feel the stretch in the middle of the back between the shoulder blades. Hold the stretch for at least 10 seconds and repeat with the other arm over the first one (see illustration on page 139).

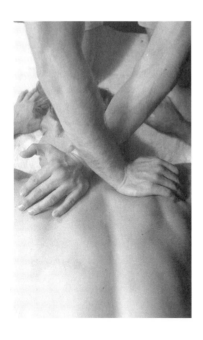

To stretch the middle back between the shoulder blades:

1. The athlete lies on his stomach with the arms to the sides or underneath the head.
2. The massager, kneeling above the head, crosses his arms and places the right hand on the inside of the right shoulder blade, the left hand is on the inside of the left shoulder blade.
3. The massager leans over the arms and pushes the shoulder blades away and down from the massager. Hold the stretch for at least 10 seconds, release the stretch, and repeat.

Massage the shoulders, back, chest, and arms of a swimmer. The massager can spend more time in one area of a muscle to help loosen the muscle or the massager can be more superficial and lightly smooth or shake the body.

Volleyball

Emphasize the legs, arms, and shoulders in the post-event massage. Work the inner and outer hips and thighs with massages and stretches for relief after doing quick lateral motion. Be loving to the shoulder and back for arms that do most of the spiking.

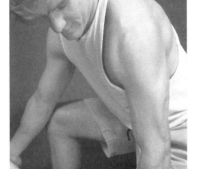

A great stretch and massage for the shoulders:

1. Start with the athlete on her back. The massager is on the left side of the athlete.
2. With his right hand, the massager brings the left arm of the athlete above the athlete's head as close to the ground as possible.
3. The massager's left hand is on the athlete's chest. It is pushing the chest muscle down to

the feet to stretch the chest more. It can also do slow shaking and jostling to relax and loosen the muscle.

The extremities are sensitive and may cramp or won't accept the muscles being massaged. The athlete's forearms may be sore or hurt from "digging" or setting balls. Slow light massage is pertinent for these areas.

Weight Lifting

A weight lifter should get the entire body, but if you are breaking the body down to body parts or areas, massage those areas. An example of this would be to lift back and biceps in one workout, in which case the massager will do post-event massage on the back and biceps. It is also good to do some compressions or kneading to the muscles between the sets. Shaking and smoothing the muscles is a must! So after the first set of bench presses, the massager would compress the chest, knead the deltoids and triceps, or shake the area for a few seconds until you start your next set. Another great one is to stretch after the massage between sets or just stretching. In the case of the bench press, stretch the chest, shoulders, and triceps, then continue with the second set. The massage will fill in the time between the sets and help you rest and rejuvenate enough to have great success in the next set. The muscles will also get the benefit of the massage. Stretch and massage the muscles that are lifting the exercise or movement. After the whole workout, the massager can just smooth, shake, or jostle the body in slow, rhythmic motions to relax the body.

Rowing and Kayaking

Rowers and kayakers use the shoulders, back, chest, wrists, and upper arms a lot. These are the areas that will be emphasized. Do post-event massage to the neck, traps, shoulders, chest, and upper arms. Just shake and smooth the legs from the hips down. While moving along, these athletes can take a break and shake out the tight muscle areas like weight lifters. Twisting movements for the torso are great to loosen and warm this vital area. Also, one may use the cramp techniques discussed in Chapter 8.

• • •

The massager and athlete must work as a team. The athlete must let the massager know where he needs the most massage. The massager helps to cool the athlete down from the competition or event. The massager also helps the athlete get more out of a stretch by increasing the range of motion of the stretch and decreasing the effort that an athlete has to expend doing these stretches. If the athlete got an injury, he must tell the massager, who will spend extra time working that area with massage. Do not do deep tissue work at the injury site, just extra massage. If there is any doubt on the pace of any of the strokes, be slow and rhythmic.

EIGHT

Maintenance and Injury Massage

In this chapter, we will go over ice massage, cramp-release techniques, and maintenance massage for important muscles and areas, both self and partner. As with any injury, see a medical doctor for the pain or serious injuries. Do not massage an injured area if the pain persists or gets worse.

Ice Massage

Ice massage is used in post-event and maintenance massage on injured, overused, and sensitive areas (trigger points, muscle attachments, injured muscle bellies, and tendons). The ice is used to reduce swelling so that you may have greater range of motion in an injured joint. Ice also slows the metabolism of the surrounding numb tissues so that less tissue dies from lack of oxygen. The tissue uses less oxygen and has less wastes built up in or around it by the decreased metabolism. The less tissue that dies, the less swelling that will occur.

Many massage therapists use cryocups bought from a massage-product dealer or school. This is great if you are going to be using it a lot. Another way is to put water into small paper cups and let it freeze. As the ice melts, just rip off the paper to reveal more of the ice. Another quicker way is to get an ice cube and put paper around the area that your fingers hold so as not to freeze your fingers.

When doing ice massage, put a towel underneath to keep area dry. When applying the ice to the skin, use small circular strokes around the area (similar to icing a cake). Do not do ice massage on areas where major nerves are superficial (the crease between the leg and hip in the front and the armpit are just two). Stop ice massage if the numbness shoots down an extremity like an arm or leg.

Ice massage is done for 5–10 minutes. During that time, the athlete will experience four phases of feelings: coldness, burning, aching, and numbness. The massager does the ice massage only until the athlete moves from the aching coldness into the fourth phase, numbness. If the massager did the ice massage longer, frostbite would occur, which is death to the tissue and a result you don't want to achieve.

Ice massage can be done by itself or after the area is massaged.

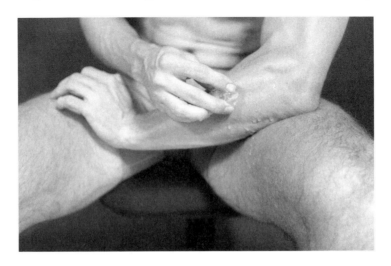

Cramp-Release Techniques

Cramp-release techniques are used to alleviate pain caused by cramps in muscles. A cramp is an involuntary contraction of a bundle of muscle fibers, which may include the entire muscle. A painful experience, cramps are caused by many different factors: loss of electrolytes or a blow to the area, to name two.

Cramps are released by stretching the affected muscle, direct pressure into the cramped muscle, a combination of stretching and pressure into the muscle, contracting the opposite muscle or muscle groups in the opposite direction of the cramp, or tapoting (repetitively striking) the muscle for an extended period of over 1 minute.

The first way we will release cramps is to stretch the muscle. For a cramp in the calves, do a calf stretch on the affected leg. The athlete should hold the stretch until the pain goes away or the cramp releases.

In the second technique, pressing into the tissue, an example for a cramp on the bottom of the foot would be to press the sole of the shoe into the edge of a sidewalk, so the sidewalk is pressing into the middle of the cramp, where it is most painful. Another way is to take off the shoe and to press your fingers into the middle of the cramp. Start the pressure light and then increase the pressure as the athlete's pain threshold will allow. Hold and breathe until the cramp releases. A massager can also grab a cramp between the thumb and fingers to pinch the affected tissue. One can also press, release the pressure, and repeat until the cramp goes away.

The third technique, the combination of stretch and press, would be done this way on a cramp in the hamstrings. The athlete with the cramp is on his back with the unaffected leg out straight and the affected leg up in the air with the hip and knee bent. The massager stretches the hamstring by bringing the knee toward the chest and presses in with an elbow or finger till the cramp goes away.

The fourth technique uses an opposite muscle group to contract and makes the target muscle group relax as the opposing muscle group contracts. If the principle did not exist, people would have a hard time walking because the quadriceps would be fighting the hamstrings, muscles in the front and back of the thigh respectively, as would other muscle groups that go against

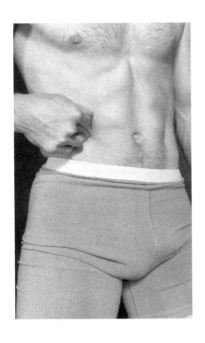

each other. Therefore, to release a cramp in the triceps muscle in the back of the arm, the biceps muscle of that arm would contract near maximally.

In the fifth technique, tapotment, an example of a cramp in the quadriceps would be to hit the area with a fist at a medium depth and a fast pace. This is done till the cramp goes away.

Another way that an athlete, a runner, say, could use these techniques will be shown on a cramp in the abdominal muscles. The cramp is painful, hard, and knotty. It makes it hard to breathe. The athlete could stop and stretch the abdominals. This is done on her stomach. She presses up the upper torso as the hips and legs stay on the ground to arch her back. She can do it to one side more than another by moving her arms to one side and leaning to that shoulder. Another way to release the cramp would be to press the tips of her fingers into the cramp as she runs. The press is held till the cramp goes away. A third method is to contract the low back muscles and lean back and away from the cramped side. She can continue to hit the area with her fist till she releases the cramp. All these techniques are easy and effective.

SELF-MAINTENANCE MASSAGE AND INJURY TREATMENT

Use the following massages as guidelines. Make them longer and use different techniques that you know. These are by no means the only massages to do for these areas. Use some of the strokes for one body part in another place. If you or your athlete are injured, remember the word RICE: Rest, Ice, Compression (*not* the stroke, but using a bandage or cloth to apply pressure to the area), and Elevation. It is important to rest the injured limb or area. Ice the area. Compress the area to avoid swelling, and elevate the limb or area to reduce the swelling.

Foot Pain

1. Take off shoes and socks for this massage.

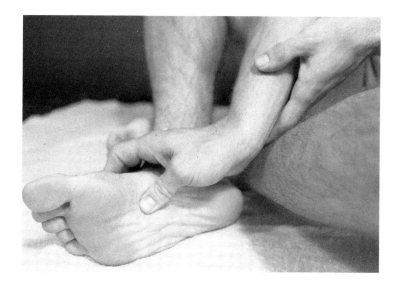

2. Sit on the ground. The right leg is straight, and the left is bent at the knee with the knee out and the foot by the right knee.

3. Warm the bottom of your left foot by smoothing with the right hand at a medium to fast pace.

4. Place the knuckles of the fist into the bottom of the foot with slow, deep strokes from heel to toes for at least 1 minute.

5. Use the fist or thumb and hold the pressure in the painful, tight tissues. Hang out with the tissue till it releases or lets go. Move slowly down from the heel to the toes. Rub or smooth the bottom of the foot to finish the area at a slow to medium pace for 20 seconds.

Acute Ankle Sprain Massage

This massage is done after the doctor has seen and diagnosed the area.

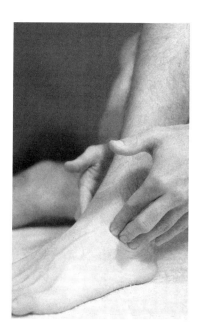

1. Warm the area above the injury area with light slow strokes that go up toward the heart.

2. Warm the area below the ankle sprain by doing the same thing: warm the area with strokes leading back to the heart.

3. Do circular ice massage onto the ankle sprained area for 5–7 minutes.

For an acute ankle sprain massage on the left ankle:
1. Start on the floor. The right leg is straight out and the left leg is bent at the knee with the left foot flat on the ground. Both palms of the hands are on the lower left leg above the ankle with the fingers pointing to the front.
2. Smooth up the leg with a stroke length of about 6–8 inches with a light touch and slow pace.
3. Increase the pressure of the stroke to light/medium-pressure smoothing leading back to the heart. Repeat these warming strokes for about 1–3 minutes.
4. Now place the palms of your hands below the injured ankle and by the toes. The left hand is on the top of the foot on the outside and the right hand is on the inside of the foot or on the bottom of the foot.
5. Smooth softly toward the body from toes to ankle. The stroke is gentle and does not cause you any pain. The left ankle is stabilized by being on the floor. Do this gentle stroking at a slow to medium pace for 1–3 minutes.
6. Finally, get an ice cube or cup and ice massage the injured ankle area till the tissue is numb, or 5–7 minutes, whichever comes first.

The purpose of the acute ankle sprain massage is to get the fluids moving through the tissues. A second reason is to ice the area to stop or remove any swelling.

Post-Acute Ankle Sprain Massage
This massage is done 24–48 hours after the injury.
1. Warm the area with smoothing that is light and does not hurt. The strokes are slow, moving up toward the heart.
2. Move the ankle through nonpainful ranges of motion. Start with just pointing the toe away from the body and then up to the body. Progress into small circles, larger circles, and then in and out (the bottom of the foot faces the inside and then the outside of the body).
3. Transverse friction the injured area to break up adhesions to achieve free range of motion.

4. Smooth and warm up the area again from toes to body. Finish with a 5-minute ice massage.

Shinsplints

1. Sit up with the left leg bent and the right leg straight. The left foot is flat on the floor and the left knee is in the air.

2. Smooth up and down the lower front leg at a medium pace with the palms of both hands. The right hand is on the bony side and the left on the muscles in front and on the outside (see top illustration on page 41).

3. Press into the inside and outside of the leg with the heels of both hands.

4. Circular compress with the heels of the hands so they move forward, down to the feet, back, up to knee, and forward again. After an area is warm and mushy, move down the leg till the strokes reach the ankle.

5. Drop the left knee sideways to the floor.

6. Reach over the leg with the fingers of the right hand and cross-fiber friction, or friction in the perpendicular direction of the muscle fibers, the areas just covered. The friction will move across the muscles that run straight down the leg. Always friction the muscles toward the crest of the bone on the inside of the lower leg (tibia).

7. Finish by smoothing the entire lower leg slowly.

Front Thigh

1. Sit in a chair and place the hand on the left quads by the knee.

2. Smooth up and down the leg till the tissues get warm.

3. Bring the hands back down to the knee area and compress the quads up to the hip with the heels of both hands at a slow to medium pace. Hold out at tight, painful areas.

4. Hold the heel of both hands into the muscles as before, but now do deep, slow circular friction with both hands. It is easier to move

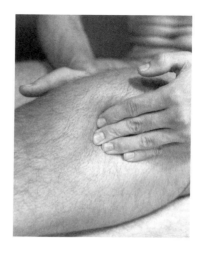

the hands together in the same direction or to move them out of sync; while one is closer to the knee, the other is closer to the hip in their small circles. Make sure to get the top of the thigh (rectus femoris) and the outside of the thigh (iliotibial band).

Groin Pulls

1. Sit on the floor with the right leg straight and the left bent. The left knee falls to the outside and the left foot is by the right knee.
2. With a loose fist of the right hand, compress the inner thigh from the hipbone down to the knee with light to medium pressure. The large muscles here love the deep holding pressure, so when you get to an injury or tight area, hold and squeeze with the heel of your hand as the pain releases or the tightness goes away.
3. Finish with compression strokes and smoothing along the entire length of the inner thigh.

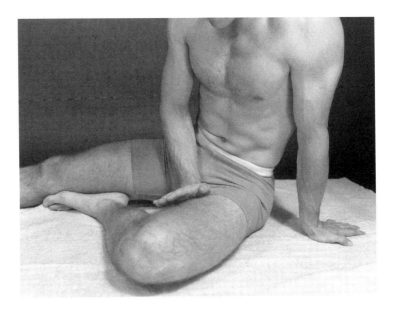

Sore Forearms

This maintenance massage is great for tennis elbow (pain on the lateral forearm), carpal tunnel syndrome, or other overuse injuries of the forearm or wrist.

1. Sit in a chair and place the forearm that will be worked on onto the corresponding leg (left forearm on the left thigh). The palm will be down.

2. Warm up the back of the forearm with kneading and compressions with the right hand. Compress with the palm of the right hand at a medium pace. Start with light pressure and increase the pressure by leaning the body into the stroke on your leg.

3. Lift the arm and knead all the forearm muscles by placing the palm heel on the front of the left arm and the fingers on the muscles in the back of the forearm.

4. Squeeze the muscles between the heel and fingers of the right hand. Knead up and down between the elbow and the wrist. Also knead the inside and outside of the forearm. Knead and compress the sore or tight muscles or tendons.

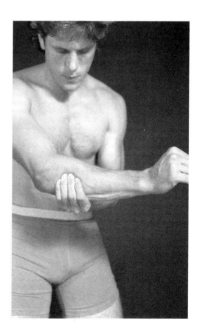

When the tight, painful areas are warm, do some cross-fiber friction on the area. The forearm muscles, generally, run up and down the forearm. So the cross-fiber friction will run back and forth across the width of the forearm.

To do the cross-fiber friction on the right arm:

1. Begin with the right hand palm down.

2. Place the left hand underneath the right forearm with the fingers just above the outside bone.

3. Press in with the fingertips of the left hand and do not move them.

4. Twist the right wrist back and forth so the palm of the right hand turns in and up. Twist the right wrist back and forth to move the

left fingers across the muscles. Do this stroke till the pain lessens, the tissue softens, or up to 5–7 minutes.

5. End by kneading or compressing the area, then smoothing the forearm in the direction of the heart.

6. Add ice massage to the areas that were the most sore.

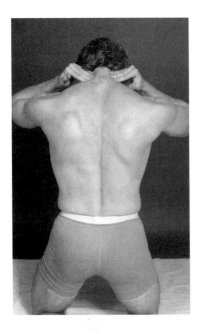

Neck

Warm up the neck by using the fingers of both hands.

1. The fingers press in on their respective sides.

2. The fingers move in small circular motions: into the spine, up to head, out, and down to the shoulders.

3. Start the massage at the area where the neck attaches to the shoulders and work your way up to where the neck joins the head.

4. Go up and down 3–4 times to warm the tissue.

5. Repeat the same stroke, but deeper. Also, hold at the tight painful areas.

6. Friction the neck with a motion across the neck: into the spine and straight out to the side.

The friction is a sawing motion. The areas just below the head and about an inch lower are great points to work on.

Traps

1. Sit in a chair and place your right hand on the muscle between the neck and shoulders.

2. The left hand grabs the right forearm at the elbow to get greater pressure with less muscle work from one arm.

3. Slowly knead the traps from the neck to the shoulder till the tissue is warm and mushy.

4. Grab the tight bands of tissue and hold them between the fingers and thumb. Hold the tight bands till they loosen or the pain subsides.

5. Press the fingers of the left hand into the muscle on the top inside edge of the shoulder blade. This is the attachment of the levator scapula muscle. Move around the area to get the most painful spot—the trigger point. Hold this area till it releases or the pain goes away.

6. Finish the area by lightly kneading the traps from neck to shoulder.

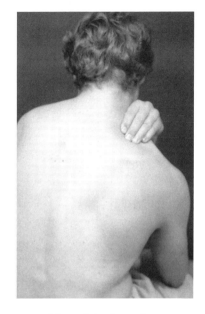

Shoulders and Upper Arm

1. Knead the left shoulder and upper arm with the right hand till the area is warm and mushy.

2. With the fingers together and the hand cupped, cross-fiber friction the deltoid from back to front.

3. Do the same to the triceps, but friction from the deltoid to the elbow.

4. For the biceps, grab the arm so the fingers are on the biceps and the thumb is on the triceps. The palm of the hand faces the inside of the upper arm but does not press into the tissue: there is a major artery that flows through this area and pressure will interrupt the blood flow (see illustration on page 51).

5. With the fingers, you will cross-fiber friction the biceps from shoulder to elbow. Massage the outer low upper arm. The muscle here, the brachialis, has a major trigger point.

Abdominals

1. Stand with the feet shoulder-width apart.

2. Place the palms of the hands on the area below the belly button.

3. Rub the entire abdominal area by going right to the side, up to the right ribs, across below the rib cage to the left side, down the left side to the hip, and back to the center below the belly button. Rub in this clockwise direction, getting the entire abdominal area.

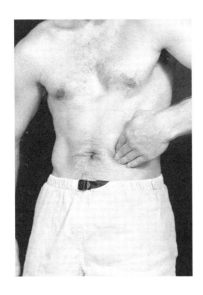

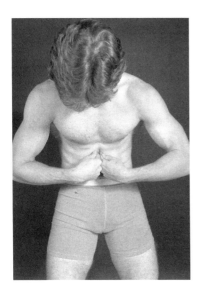

4. Using the tips of your fingers, press in both sides with the same hand and circular friction the entire area.

5. Put the backs of both hands together with the wrist and hand bent.

Here, too, remember to avoid the xiphoid provess. When working by the abdominals, avoid the upper area by the solar plexus. The bone tapers off to a small process called the xiphoid process. This process can break off and puncture the diaphragm.

6. Press into the abdominals up below the solar plexus (avoid the lower sternum) with the tips of the fingers. Make sure that you are about two fingers' width below where the ribs join in the center of the chest. As you press into the abdominals, breathe out and bend your body slightly forward to release the stretch on the abdominals.

7. Move your fingers to the left halfway to the edge of your body and repeat. Breathe in, then breathe out and press in with the fingertips of both hands.

8. Move to the edge of the left abdominals by the rib cage and repeat.

9. Move down to just above the left hip and repeat.

10. Move halfway into the center of the hip and repeat.

11. Repeat now at the center above the hip, to halfway to the right, to the right, to the right at the rib cage, halfway to the center, and back to the center. The pressure of this technique is not too deep. The abdominals lie above the internal organs. If you go too deep or too fast, you could hurt one of them.

12. Lean back slightly and friction the entire abdominal area with the tips of your fingers. Remember to breathe in and out as you do the frictioning. If you get to a tight or painful area, take a deep breath in to get deeper pressure on the muscle. This is better than pressing in with the fingers because the breath will extend the abdominal muscles.

Chest

1. Stand with feet shoulder-width apart.
2. Place the right heel of the hand on your left chest. *For women, avoid the breast tissue area.* It is the chest muscle we are working.
3. Smooth the area with the right hand from the center of the chest to the shoulder. Feel the muscle stretching out.
4. Press the heel of the right hand into the tissue in compression strokes. Massage the areas below the collarbone (clavicle) to the shoulder, to the nipple, to the breastbone (sternum), up to the collarbone.
5. Place the tips of the fingers into the pectoral muscles and circular friction the area in small circular strokes. Hold out at tight areas to loosen them up.
6. Finish by rubbing or smoothing the left pectoral.

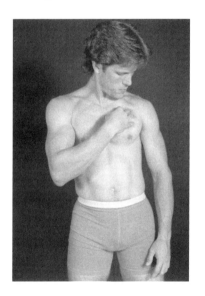

Lower Back

1. Lie on the right side.
2. Smooth the left low back area with the left hand till the tissue is warm.
3. Make a fist with the left hand and place the back of the knuckles into the muscles right next to the spine on the left side. Knuckle the areas between the ribs and the hips, from the spine to the outside of the body (love-handle area).

4. Put the fingers together straight out and press the ends of the fingers into the side of the muscles next to the spine on the left side.

5. Press in and friction the area. The direction is from head to toe (longitudinal friction). Press and hold in the tight, painful area.

6. Finish by rubbing the area with the heel of the left hand.

Back

The muscles by the spine in the back are hard to reach by yourself. The massage businesses have created many tools to get at these areas. Things like a massage cane or wooden dowels, knobs, or balls all work great. You could even use a tennis ball. To get these areas (except the cane versions that can be used while standing), it is best to lie on the piece of equipment and relax till the tension or pain goes away. These objects can also be used by placing them between a wall and yourself, but you won't be using all your weight to push the object into the muscle. So for the back, it is best to get a massage tool and lie on your back or to get someone else to massage it.

PARTNER MAINTENANCE MASSAGE

Foot

1. The athlete is lying on her stomach, barefooted.

2. Kneel by her feet, facing toward her head. (Keep your inside knee on the ground and your outside leg with its knee in the air and the foot on the ground. This will help you to get leverage to press into the tissue without overusing your muscles.)

3. Starting with light pressure, knuckle down the foot from the heel to the toes with a loose fist and light pressure.

4. After the tissue is nice and warm, press the thumb (or finger or one knuckle) into the base of the heel. Get the middle, outside, and inside of the heel. Press in and hold the pressure for at least 15 seconds, then release slowly. Repeat till the pain goes away or the tight area loosens, or move to the other areas of the heel.

5. Another great area that needs digital pressure is the heel on the inside edge, just off the bone. Again press into it with the thumb and hold for at least 15 seconds.

6. Repeat if necessary.
7. Finish by smoothing the entire bottom of the foot with light, slow strokes.

Another great area to work on the foot is the top of the foot between each bone, just above where the toes connect to the foot. The muscles in here help hold the foot together and stabilize the forces of contact as the foot holds the body up during walking.

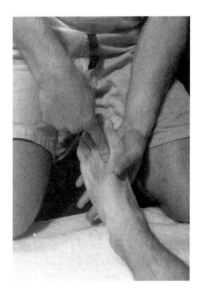

1. Just press into the spaces between the toe bones with a thumb or braced finger and hold the pressure or do circular frictioning for at least 15 seconds.
2. Repeat again if necessary or move on to the next toe.

1. The athlete is on her stomach, barefooted.
2. The massager is by her feet.
3. Rub the feet with the palms to warm the tissue.
4. Press into the bottom of the foot with a loose fist.
5. Compress and friction the area with the fist.
6. Press the bottom of the foot with the thumb in straight lines. Hold and compress the tight, painful spots.
7. End by smoothing with the fist from heel to toes.

Lower Leg and Ankle
1. The athlete is on his back.
2. The massager is kneeling by his feet.
3. Compress the outside lower leg with the heel of your hands.
4. After you warm the tissue, press your thumbs into the muscle in all directions, and "walk" the thumbs up and down the muscles in a straight line from knee to ankle.

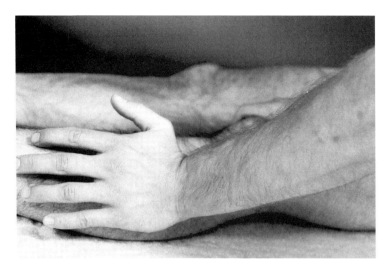

5. Friction the whole area from knee to ankle with the pads of your fingertips in slow, deep frictions.
6. Finish with compressions.

Front Thigh

1. The athlete is on her back, legs out straight.
2. The massager is on the right side of the leg that is being massaged between the hip and knee.
3. Compress the quadriceps with the heel of the hands.
4. Knead them.
5. Friction the area in straight lines and get the areas that are designated as great to get (at the end of the chapter).
6. Finish by smoothing the entire top area from hip to knee.

Hamstrings

1. The athlete is on his stomach, legs out straight.
2. The massager is on the side of the leg to be worked on, between the knee and the hip.
3. Compress with the heel of your hand up and down the muscles. Hold the compressions at the tight, knotty spots and move the heel in circles as you continue the pressure (see top illustration on page 111).
4. Finish by smoothing the entire area.

Groin Area

1. The athlete is lying on her left side with the left leg straight out and the right leg bent at the hip and knee. The right knee is on the ground. Her left arm is over her head with the head resting on the upper arm, or the arm is bent with the left hand underneath the head. The right arm is in front of the body with the hand resting on the floor.

2. The massager faces the same direction the athlete faces. The massager will be between the knee and the butt behind her.

3. Make a fist and place onto the inner thigh area on the straight, exposed bottom leg. One of the hands will be the massaging hand and the other will sit and stabilize you as you lean into the strokes. It does not matter which hand is used—the movement and stabilizing hand may also switch.

4. Compress into the inner thigh area starting from the butt to the knee with light pressure. The first adductor that must loosen is the gracilis muscle: the thin, long muscle that is the most superficial. It lies right in the middle of the inner thigh.

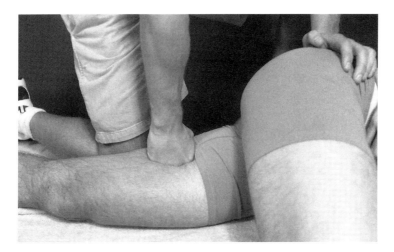

5. Once this muscle loosens, apply deeper pressure to get the other adductors. Work the back and the front of the inner thigh. When you get to an area that is painful or tight, all you have to do is hold the compression and sink your weight into it. Hold the pressure for at least 15 seconds, release slowly, and repeat till it loosens up.

6. Finish the area by compressing or kneading the inner thigh.

Butt

1. The athlete is on his stomach with the arms at his sides and the legs out straight.
2. The massager is at the hip area facing the opposite shoulder from the side of the butt that you want to work on. If the massager is on the right side, the right hand does the compressions.
3. Twist the compression into the butt with your fists. Start from the inside, just off the middle of the butt bone (the sacrum).

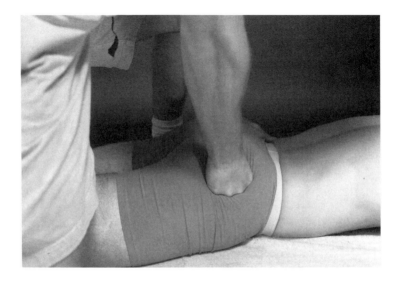

4. Compress to the outside by the side of the hip. Move down the butt.
5. Massage the entire side of the butt by going in circles and straight lines. Hold at the tight trigger points.
6. Finish the area by smoothing in circles or shaking the area vigorously.

Lower Back

1. The athlete is on her stomach, arms by her sides and the legs out straight.
2. The massager is on the opposite side of the back that is going to be worked on.
3. With the palm of one hand (the other is held stationary around the area), compress right along the opposite side of the low back. Compress

down and up the erector muscles from the bottom of the ribs to the top of the hips. Hold the compressions on the trigger-point areas.

4. Stretch the lower back (shown in the postevent partner massage — see illustration on page 150) by taking the top hand and pressing the top of the hip down. The bottom hand crosses the other arm and presses up on the back by the ribs. Hold the stretch for at least 10 seconds.

5. Move to the same side of the low back that you are working on.

6. Do circular compressions at the edge of the lower back muscles about 3 inches away from the spine. Hold the tight, painful areas.

7. Place both palms of your hands on the sacrum.

8. Press the sacrum down to the floor and to the feet. This decompresses the lower back and feels great. Hold the stretch for at least 10 seconds.

9. Finish the area by shaking it vigorously or smoothing down from the ribs to the hips.

Back

1. The athlete is on his stomach, arms by his sides and the legs out straight.

2. The massager is on the opposite side of the back being worked on.

3. Compress the other side of the back with the palm of one hand while the other stays stationary. Get the area from the neck to the hips at least 3 times. Hold the compressions on the tight areas.

4. Move to the same side of the back that you are working on and press in on the muscles on the shoulder blade.

5. Do circular compressions and holding of those compression. Compress the area from the inside edge of the shoulder blade to the outside of the shoulder.

6. Move above the shoulders and head.

7. Compress down on the top of the trapezius muscle on the same side you are working on. Hold the compressions on the tight areas and at the top inside of the shoulder blade (see illustration on page 106).

8. Finish the back by compressing the entire area at a slower pace.

Shoulder

1. The athlete is lying on her stomach, her face pointing to one side. The arm on that side sits out from the shoulder, and bent up at a 90-degree angle. The other arm is straight down by her side.
2. Lean on one side or straddle over her.
3. Place the heels of your hands onto the muscles in the back of her shoulder blade.
4. Press in and move the shoulder blades in circular motions. Repeat this as you watch the muscles relax and loosen.
5. Press the shoulder blade into the ribs gently. Increase the pressure slowly if needed by leaning onto your arms. This will work through the shoulder base and get the muscle underneath it: the subscapularis. Hold for at least 15 seconds and repeat on another area of the shoulder blade. Do not work through the bumpy crest of the shoulder blade, for this will cause pain. Stay below the crest and work in and out and at different angles to get other areas of the subscapularis muscle (see illustration on page 107).
6. Straddled above her, move to one side of her body. Work on the side opposite the raised arm and face. When you change sides, have the athlete change her head and arm to be opposite your working side again.
7. Kneel on the opposite leg and face her body with the front of your body angled up to their head.
8. Place the inside heel of your right hand above the top inner part of the shoulder blade between the shoulder blade and the neck.
9. Compress the muscles on the top inner edge of the shoulder blade with the heel of the hand. (The hand is turned so the outside heel of the hand is doing the compression, not the whole heel of the hand.) Compress the muscles with the heel of your hand down the inner edge of the shoulder blade and below the lower inside edge. It is easiest to have the hand turned so the fingers are across the body toward the other shoulder blade as you go down the inner edge. The left hand is resting on the other left shoulder with little to no weight on it.
10. Move the left hand so that it cups the front of her left shoulder, your other hand on her back.

11. Push the shoulder into the body and up so the shoulder blade rises off the back. The inside shoulder-blade muscles have to be loose to do this, so loosen them up with more compressions if the shoulder blade still seems tight. With the right hand, grab underneath the inside edge of the shoulder blade and pull it up and away from the back slightly. She will feel a stretch into the neck and a release. It feels great!

12. Slowly release the inner edge of the shoulder blade as you lower it. Keep the right hand on the muscles between the shoulder blade and the spine. The left will compress into the outer edge of the shoulder blade muscles below the armpit.

13. Compress with the outer edge of the heel of your hand.

14. Knead the shoulder muscle, the deltoid, with the left hand. Massage the front and the back of the deltoid.

15. Stretch the shoulder again. Your left hand stays in front of the athlete's left shoulder, your right grabs the athlete's left arm by the inside elbow. Lift the arm off the ground slightly and pull the arm down the body. Hold the stretch for at least 10 seconds.

16. With the arm off the ground, rotate the left shoulder in circles: up, forward, down, back. Do at least 3 circles, repeat the same number in the opposite direction, and then knead the area.

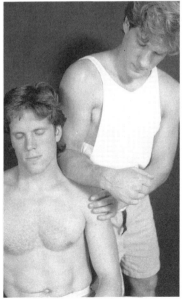

17. Finish by holding the shoulder lightly to the ground.

Traps

1. The athlete is sitting on a chair.

2. Move to the athlete's back left side and place the end of your right forearm by the elbow on the muscle between the neck and the left shoulder. Place the end of your elbow into the belly of the left traps.

3. Lean onto the forearm to get pressure and give slow compression strokes. Start at a light depth

and work deeper. Massage a triangle area from the neck down to the top of the inside shoulder blade and out to the shoulder. Compress the areas till the traps gets nice and soft.

4. Press into the middle of the traps where it is at its thickest and hold. As you hold the pressure, ask the athlete to drop her head to the right front part of her shoulder, away from you. Ask her if she feels the stretch all the way up her neck. Hold the stretch for at least 10 seconds.

5. Bring her head back to neutral.

6. Compress some more with the end of your forearm.

7. Move to the other side by kneading both the left and right traps with your respective hands for about 1 minute. Finish the transition by smoothing both the traps muscles with the palms of both hands.

8. Put the hands next to the neck and slide them to the shoulder. Take off the pressure and repeat 2 more times.

9. Move to the right side of her shoulder in the back and repeat. Make sure that she is sitting straight and breathing. Do not let her slouch or hold her breath.

Abdominals

1. The athlete is lying on his back. If the athlete has a shirt on, have him take it off or just raise the shirt to rib level in the middle of the body where the ribs meet the sternum.

2. Move to one side of the abdominals—the side that is most comfortable to you.

3. Place the palms of your hands on the middle of his abdominals just below the rib cage.

4. Smooth the entire abdominal area by going in a clockwise, circular path. Move the palms of your hands to his left, down to the left hip, across the bottom to the right hip, up to the right ribs, and back across the middle. Repeat this circle 5 times. The hands can move together or alternate. If the hands alternate and you are on the athlete's right side, the right hand is closer to the hip and the left is closer to the ribs. The right (lower) hand does not leave the body. The left (upper) hand lifts over the right hand when it is at the lower middle part of the abdominals

and the right is at the upper middle part of the abdominals. After the hand slides over the other, it returns to the abdominals.

5. Place the heels of the hands on the nearest side of the rectus abdominal (the middle abdominal muscle) and the fingers on the other side of the muscle. The hands are together.

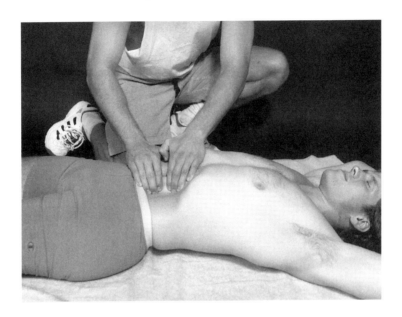

6. Move the muscle back and forth by pulling and pushing the muscle in a stroking motion. Feel the muscle loosen and have greater movement.

7. Gently press into the lower, middle abdominals just above the pelvis bone. The hands are angled down toward the legs.

8. Slowly friction back and forth across the body with transverse friction. Friction for at least 20 seconds only in the middle of the abdominals. If you move out to either side and press in, you will be pressing on major arteries and nerves. That is a no-no.

9. Place the tips of the fingers into the abdominal area. The fingers are spread so they look like a rake.

10. With the tips of your fingers, circular friction all the abdominals. Hold and friction for at least 5 seconds, release the pressure, move the hands somewhere else, and continue till the entire abdominal area is done. Be

careful of the sides of the lower abdominal by the pelvis bone and the top middle of the abdominals where the ribs meet the sternum.

11. Finish by smoothing in a clockwise circle the entire abdominals area with the palms of your hands, as when we started the abdominal massage.

Chest

1. The athlete is on his back with the legs out straight.
2. The massager is on the side he will be massaging.
3. Move the arm on the side you are on so that it is open to about 90 degrees (nearly straight out to the side). Kneel by the hip between the arm and the body. Face toward the head.
4. If you are on the left side of the body and thus working the left chest, press your right palm into the chest muscle just off the sternum. *On women, you do not work the breast tissue* (see illustration on page 115).
5. Compress the chest muscle in straight lines from inside to the shoulder. Also compress in circles. The depth and pace is medium. After the tissue is warm, press the top, inside, lower, and outside of the chest muscles with your thumbs.
6. Friction the tissue away and toward the center of the chest. Then friction the chest in straight lines.
7. Finish the area with compressions and then shaking the tissue at a quicker pace and lighter depth then the initial strokes.

Upper Arm

1. The athlete is on his back with the arms to the side and the legs out straight.
2. The massager is on the same side as the arm being massaged. Kneel around the shoulder on the outside of the arm.
3. Bring the athlete's hand onto his stomach and kneel below his elbow to hold the arm in place.
4. Knead the front upper arm with both hands.
5. Stop and then compress the biceps muscle with your inside arm, the arm closest to the athlete's body. Hold the compressions to work the tissue.

6. With your other (outside) hand, knead the shoulder muscle, the deltoid.

7. After the muscle is warm, muscle strip (use your thumbs to make long straight lines up and down the muscle) the muscle from a point on the outside of the upper arm up to the inside, middle, and back of the shoulder.

8. Lift the athlete's hand to the top of the same shoulder.

9. Move to the shoulder area of his body and face the arm and other shoulder.

10. Knead the back of the upper arm muscle, the triceps, with both hands.

11. Stop and then move to the top of his body and face the feet.

12. Muscle strip the triceps muscle with both thumbs from elbow to shoulder. Massage the inside, middle, and outside of the upper, back arm.

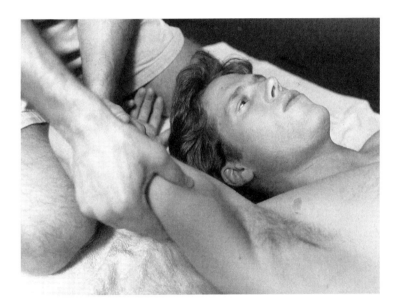

13. Finish the upper arm by lowering it to the ground straight and shaking the areas worked on.

Forearm

1. The athlete is on his back with the arms to the side and the legs out straight.

2. The massager is on the same side as the arm being massaged. Kneel around the forearm. The athlete's palm is facing the front.

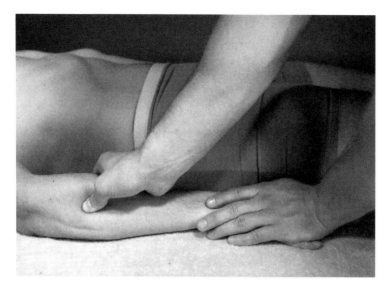

3. Compress the top of the forearm (the wrist extensor muscles) with the palm of your outside hand. Compress the area from the bottom of the elbow to the wrist. Hold the compression on any sore areas.
4. Muscle strip (see the upper arm above) in straight lines in the same area.
5. Finish with lighter compression.
6. Turn the arm over so the inside of the forearm is showing (the palm is up).
7. Compress the wrist flexor muscles with the palm of your inside hand from the inside of the elbow to the wrist. Hold the compressions on the tight areas.
8. Muscle strip the area.
9. Finish with lighter compressions than before.

Hand
1. The athlete is on his back with the arms to the side and the legs out straight. The palms are down.
2. The massager is on the same side as the arm being massaged. Kneel around the hand to be massaged.
3. Grab the hand with both hands so your fingers are on the palm and the thumbs point toward the wrist.
4. Squeeze the hand so that the hand spreads and your fingers move to the outside.

5. Do this at least 3 times, then friction the top back of the hand between the fingers (the metacarpal bone area).

6. Grab the hand as before and make the hand move in waves as you mobilize and stretch the hand.

7. Turn the hand over and friction the muscles on the thumb and little finger, palm side. Hold the tight painful areas.

8. Finish with the technique that you started with: spreading the palm of the hand.

Neck

1. The athlete is sitting on a chair, arms at his sides.

2. The massager is at the top of the head facing the feet.

3. Stand behind the head with the tip of your fingers pressed into the neck at the bottom of the head.

4. Press in and just hold the tension on these very important muscles.

5. Friction slightly with both hands in circles. Move your hand down the neck about a half of an inch and press in. There is a great spot here where a few muscles cross each other.

6. Finish by circular frictioning lightly up and down the back of the neck with one hand on the one side and then the other hand on the other side.

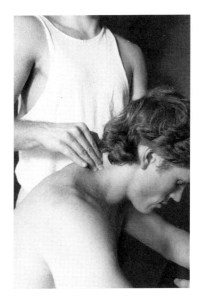

We have now done the entire body, both self and partner massages. Try out these techniques. Use these great maintenance massages to help relieve tension and get rid of the knots. In the bibliography are some other books that will help you get more experience in massages and change your massages. All this and more will help your body be better prepared for your activity or sport.

NINE

The Art of Touch

In this day and age of AIDS, herpes, and other terrible diseases, many people fear touch and touching another. Touch may be too sexual or intimate; it can also be brutal or insensitive. But it can also be caring. When you touch and do massage on someone or yourself, you can bring back memories and emotions. The experience of our life is stored in our bodies. One must have the highest ideals when doing massage: to help another person. With education and care (see Chapter 3), massage is safe, fun, and beneficial for everyone, especially the athlete.

To get further information, contact local massage therapists, local massage schools, or organizations that publish massage material. To augment what you have learned in this book, look to related areas like stretching, sports performance, general or sports massage books, yoga, hypnosis, meditation, and exercise. To get a massage, find therapists through friends, health-food or bookstores, the yellow pages, or massage schools. Ask to see their licenses and certifications. Ask about their education, experience, and references—sport teams and private clients. Ask them about their interests, specialties, how long the massage will be, what type of massages they give, and the price of the massage. Do not settle for anything less than what you want.

I would like to finish by reemphasizing the importance of massage, one human being touching another. Scientifically massage works by warming up tissue, loosening tissue, and increasing circulation. No matter how great the massage therapist or body worker, it is the body that does the healing. We must always keep this in mind. Because of the huge amount of skin and skin receptors (light touch, deep pressure, pain, hot-cold, etc.) on our skin, and the importance of the skin as the physical border that holds us in and separates us from others, touch is a powerful therapy. It shows connection, support, and love. It is this task and responsibility that you undertake in touching a human being.

EXERCISE

1: Ask yourself what did you want to get from this book? Write your answer down at the bottom of the page.

2: Skim through the entire book from beginning to end. Before skimming, ask yourself what you wanted out of this book. Take five minutes to look at the chapter headings, pictures, diagrams, and the different sports. Keep your "what you want" in focus.

3: Close your eyes and imagine yourself doing sports massage on yourself and athletes. See, feel, touch, hear, smell, taste the movie of your massage in your mind as you do this. You are doing the massages and techniques perfectly. You or the athletes are getting the most out of the massage.

4: Do a routine in the book for the sport that you—or the athletes that you are massaging—are doing, in your mind. Picture this massage in the same way as in # 3.

5: End the inner movies with a feeling of being happy and content with what you have learned and experienced in this book and in sports massage.

Acknowledgments

I thank my editor, Mauro DiPreta, at HarperCollins for believing in me.

I thank John Wehr for getting me started in massage. I thank Marla Chefetz and Morgan Richardson for giving me my start in the real world of New York City personal training. I thank Greg Serdahl for his confidence in me and for giving me opportunities to practice massage on athletes. I thank Liz Oliver, Carol Espel, Donna Olson, TDB, Geralyn Coopersmith, and all the other great trainers and staff at the old Apex studio for a delightful experience. I thank all my clients at Sports Training Institute, Apex, and the U.S. Athletic Training Center—especially Diane Reverand. I thank the owners of the U.S. Athletic Training Center: Gary and Mary Guerriero. I thank Alex Goelet for giving me great experiences in training and massage. I thank Bill and Ann Ziff for an excellent opportunity. I thank my friends, family, the Skaars, Craig, Chris, Dad, and Mom. I thank my wife, Jane, for her patience.

I especially thank a great friend: Doug Stumpf. Without him, this book definitely would not have been conceived, written, or published.

Bibliography

Alter, M. J. *Sport Stretch.* Champaign, Ill.: Leisure Press, 1990.

Anderson, B. *Stretching.* Bolinas, Calif.: Shelter, 1980.

Ashley, M. *Massage, A Career At Your Fingertips.* Bradley Beach, N.J.: Enterprise Publishing, 1992.

Benjamin, P. J., and S. P. Lamp. *Understanding Sports Massage.* Champaign, Ill.: Human Kinetics, 1996.

Daniels, L. and C. Worthingham. *Muscle Testing: Techniques of Manual Examination.* Philadelphia, Pa.: W. B. Saunders Company, 1986.

Downing, G. *The Massage Book.* New York, N.Y.: Random House, 1972.

Fahey, T. D. *Athletic Training: Principles and Practice.* Mountain View, Calif.: Mayfield Publishing Company, 1986.

Johnson, J. *The Healing Art of Sports Massage.* Emmaus, Pa.: Rodale Press, 1995.

Juhan, D. *Job's Body: A Handbook for Bodywork.* Barrytown, N.Y.: Station Hill Press, 1987.

King, R. K. *Performance Massage.* Champaign, Ill.: Human Kinetics, 1993.

Knight, K. L. *Cryotherapy in Sport Injury Management.* Champaign, Ill.: Human Kinetics, 1995.

Lundberg, P. *The Book of Shiatzu.* New York, N.Y.: Fireside, 1992.

Magee, D. J. *Orthopedic Physical Assessment.* Philadelphia, Pa.: W. B. Saunders Company, 1987.

McAtee, R. E. *Facilitated Stretching.* Champaign, Ill.: Human Kinetics, 1993.

Meagher, J. *Sportsmassage.* Barrytown, N.Y.: Station Hill Press, 1990.

Montgomery, K. *Sports Touch®: The Athletic Ritual.* San Diego, Calif.: Sports Touch®, 1990.

Tappan, F. M. *Healing Massage Techniques: Holistic, Classic, and Emerging Methods.* Norwalk, Conn.: Appleton & Lange, 1988.

Taylor, P. M., and D. K. Taylor. *Conquering Athletic Injuries.* Champaign, Ill.: Human Kinetics, 1988.

Tobias, M., and J. P. Sullivan. *Complete Stretch.* New York, N.Y.: Alfred A. Knopf, 1994.

Tortora, G. *Principles of Anatomy and Physiology.* New York, N.Y.: HarperCollins College Publishers, 1993.

White, T. P. *The Wellness Guide to Lifelong Fitness.* New York, N.Y.: Rebus, 1993.

Wood, E. C., and P. D. Becker. *Beard's Massage.* Philadelphia, Pa.: W. B. Saunders Company, 1981.